LIVING WITH BRAIN INJURY

A Guide for Families and Caregivers

Edited by Sonia Acorn and Penny Offer

An injury to the brain can affect every aspect of a person's daily life, including physical abilities and psychological make-up, relationships and family roles, school and employment, recreation and leisure. At the hospital, you may hear a lot about brain injury but not realize the importance of what you've learned until you have to deal with the injured person at home. In this handy reference book, health-care and legal experts from Canada and the United States guide you through the process of rehabilitation and help you learn how to live with brain injury. The advice of these professionals is complemented by the stories of two people who have survived injuries and are adjusting to their new lives.

Editors

SONIA ACORN is Associate Professor and Associate Director, Academic Programs, in the School of Nursing at the University of British Columbia.

PENNY OFFER is Director of the Adolescents/Young Adults Program at the G.F. Strong Rehabilitation Centre in Vancouver, British Columbia.

Living with Brain Injury

A Guide for Families and Caregivers

Edited by Sonia Acorn and Penny Offer

UNIVERSITY OF TORONTO PRESS
Toronto Buffalo London

© University of Toronto Press Incorporated 1998
Toronto Buffalo London
Printed in Canada

ISBN 0-8020-4265-1 (cloth)
ISBN 0-8020-8103-7 (paper)

Printed on acid-free paper

Canadian Cataloguing in Publication Data

Main entry under title:

Living with brain injury : a guide for families and caregivers

Includes bibliographical references.
ISBN 0-8020-4265-1 (bound)   ISBN 0-8020-8103-7 (pbk.)

1. Brain damage – patients – Rehabilitation.   2. Brain damage – patients –
Family relationships.   I. Acorn, Sonia Griffin.   II. Offer, Penny.

RC387.5.L58 1998   362.1'97481   C98-930865-0

University of Toronto Press acknowledges the financial assistance to its
publishing program of the Canada Council for the Arts and the Ontario
Arts Council.

This book is dedicated to the many individuals and their families living with the impact of a brain injury. They have inspired the editors and the authors to give their time and energy to the creation of this guide for other families and caregivers.

Any proceeds from the publication of this book will be used by the editors for education and research in brain injury.

Contents

LIVING WITH BRAIN INJURY

1. Introduction

Penny Offer, MSW, MPA

If you are like most people, you don't think very much about your brain and its miraculous ability to enable you to do everything you do – moving, talking, planning, and reacting appropriately, to name only a few of people's daily activities. Until, if you are unlucky, you are told that you, a loved one, or friend has had a brain injury. It often takes months or even years before you truly understand what this means and how it will affect the rest of your life. The brain is a very complex structure that is not fully understood. This means that every brain injury is different, and every situation unique.

This book is for *you* – for the family member or friend who must now provide some care for, or live with, or simply know, a person with a brain injury. In the days and weeks following the injury you will hear and learn much about brain injury. You will also likely forget much of this information in the turmoil of that initial time. Also, you may not understand the importance of some of the things you are told until you realize that the person has changed and you have to deal with a variety of new behaviours. While much of this book focuses on traumatic brain injury, it is equally applicable to brain injury that results from causes other than a 'blow to the head,' such as stroke, loss of oxygen, or a tumour. The causes of the injury are not as important as the injury's location in the brain, and its extent (see chapter 2). This book talks about survivor and family needs following discharge from acute medical care, and what to expect in rehabilitation, and adjusting to life after brain injury.

We hope this book will be a useful reference for you as you journey into the unknown world of brain injury. We will touch on many aspects of brain injury that will be of concern to you. We have tried to present the material in language that is easy to understand, and to provide some practical ideas and understanding of what it is like to have a brain injury. We hope you will find it useful to pick up this book from time to time, to refer to when faced with a new aspect of brain injury. In chapter 8, David Blanche describes his brain injury as his constant companion – his albatross. He talks about how he struggled for 'normality' following his brain injury. He searched and searched, and finally, after many years, when he thought he was again close to normality, he realized it was an illusion. In chapter 3, Charles Ottewell, another survivor, talks about the importance of succeeding – at being able to accomplish a task. In chapter 9, David Seaton, a psychologist from Texas, recognizes this need and the role that achieving successes plays in fostering self-esteem and motivation.

This book is written for both Canadian and American readers. Though many of the issues are the same on both sides of the border, we address specific topics in ways that recognize some of the differences in the two health care systems. In chapter 13, Brian Webster, a Canadian lawyer, offers information on the legal implications of brain injury as they apply in the United States. The financial and legal systems in both countries are quite different; within each country there are often significant differences from state to state and province to province. We do not attempt to give you all the details of these systems. Rather, we try to give you information and ideas about what to be aware of, what questions to ask, and where you might obtain additional information.

The authors include both American and Canadian representatives who are well known, sometimes in both countries, for their work in brain injury rehabilitation. All the authors are committed to making a difference in the life of brain injury survivors and their families. Some people believe that for a person with a brain injury, life and rehabilitation are the same thing – that after a while rehabilitation *becomes* life, which is a process of continuing growth. An example: Over the years, because of problems with his gait, David Blanche did a lot of falling, and eventually he learned to fall without hurting himself. He is now very athletic, hiking and biking. His ability to fall without hurting himself has helped him tremendously in his athletic endeavours, which are now a key part of his life.

The book addresses many aspects of life that are affected by an injury to the brain, including physical abilities, relationships, psychological changes, family roles, school and employment, and recreation and leisure. Because the brain plays a vital role in every aspect of daily living, a brain injury will have a profound impact on survivors and their families. Many of the chapters talk about how the individual becomes a totally different person after the injury, and offer suggestions for adjusting to this new individual. Chapter 15 stresses the need to look after yourself, to continue your own life as you adjust to the changes around you.

Brain injuries have been called a 'silent epidemic' in both Canada and the United States. The actual incidence of brain injury is unknown because accurate reporting systems are not in place. That being said, studies in both countries have begun to give us a picture of the enormity of the problem. One recent document from British Columbia, Canada (*Restoring Hope*, by Dr John Higenbottam, 1994), indicates that the rate of traumatic brain injury in that province is 150 cases per 100,000. Similar rates have been suggested for other areas. A 1991 study in the United States, 'Brain Injury in Santa Clara County' indicates that the incidence of traumatic brain injury for that county in that year was 126.9 per 100,000, and that for acquired brain injury the rate was 292.9 per 100,000. Several of the authors discuss the epidemic of brain injury in North America, and how the epidemic has changed in complexity with advances in medical technology and in prevention.

This book does not attempt to quantify the extent of brain injury. More accurate figures in each jurisdiction would help support an ideal plan for rehabilitation and long-term support and care for individuals with a brain injury. However, we know that many individuals and their families are forced to cope with little or no support after the initial phases of acute medical intervention and rehabilitation. While the numbers are interesting and certainly shocking, for the purposes of this book we have focused on those aspects of the silent epidemic that affect the day-to-day life of survivors and their families. We have attempted to provide basic information about brain injury that will help you understand and deal with the new, often frustrating, and often stressful results of a brain injury in someone you know and love. We believe that there is hope. The contributions of Charles Ottewell and David Blanche show that there is.

In our work in the field of brain injury in British Columbia over a number of years, we spoke with many families and friends seeking information and understanding about brain injury. Besides understanding, they sought advice and guidance to help them deal with this sudden and dramatic change in their lives. It seemed to us that there was a need for a handy and useful guide that would focus on what comes after the acute, medical phase of recovery – for a reference book, easy to read and readily available, that would provide information and guidance for the long journey through the unknown world of brain injury. We hope the information and ideas in this book, and the remarkable personal stories of Charles Ottewell and David Blanche, will offer you hope.

2. What Is a Brain Injury?

John Higenbottam, PhD

What is a brain injury? Is there a difference between a head injury and a brain injury? Can people be born with a brain injury? Are the effects of brain injury temporary or permanent? What are mild, moderate, and severe brain injury? Do you have to lose consciousness to have a brain injury?

Most importantly, in this chapter we will answer a number of key questions about what brain injury *means* – to you, to your family and friends, and to society.

Acquired Brain Injury

Brain injury happens when the brain's tissue is damaged or is not able to function properly. Anything that can damage brain tissue can cause a brain injury. Many brain injuries are the result of a blow to the head – that is, they are 'traumatic.' Traumatic injury may result from a fall, a sports injury, an assault, or a cycling or motor vehicle accident. In younger people, cycling and motor vehicle accidents are responsible for most cases of brain injury.

However, there are many ways in which the brain may be injured without a blow to the head. Examples: the brain can lose its blood supply, or a blood vessel can break so that bleeding into brain tissue occurs. This type of brain injury is commonly referred to as 'stroke.' Stroke is one of the most frequent causes of brain injury in older adults.

The brain may also be injured through a drug overdose, a tumour, an infection, an excess supply of protective fluid (cerebral spinal fluid), or a lack of oxygen. Whatever the type of injury, the problems and needs of survivors, their families, and caregivers are often the same. So it is important to focus on the survivor's needs and rehabilitation rather than on what caused the brain injury. This explains why the term 'acquired brain injury' is now becoming popular.

Acquired brain injury is an impairment of normal brain function due to head injury, stroke, bleeding into the space between the brain and the skull, loss of oxygen, tumours, and other diseases of the brain. Most often, brain injury that occurred before or during birth or that is due to genetic factors is not considered to be acquired brain injury.

The term 'head injury' has also been used to refer to brain injury. It is argued that this term is more acceptable because 'brain injury' implies abnormal behaviour. Unfortunately, the term 'head injury' is not always accurate, since it includes many other injuries to the head – such as those to the cheek, and jaw or skull fractures – that may not involve the brain.

In this book we are concerned with injuries to the brain and will be referring to these as 'brain injuries' or 'acquired brain injuries.'

How Often Does a Brain Injury Occur?

Brain injury is the great 'silent epidemic' of our times. It is generally agreed that for traumatic brain injury alone, there are 150 new cases a year per 100,000 people. This means that in Canada, 56,000 new cases occur each year. (In the United States there are 500,000 new cases each year.)

Of these cases, 9,000 Canadians (and 80,000 Americans) will have significant long-term rehabilitation needs.

These figures apply only to *traumatic* brain injury. The number of *acquired* brain injury survivors is much larger, since these include people for whom the brain injury is the result of a stroke, a disease, a drug overdose, or some other nontraumatic event.

Since so many cases of brain injury are due to cycling and motor vehicle accidents, haven't seat belts and helmets made a difference?

Certainly they have. However, while they may be decreasing the number of cases of traumatic brain injury, improvements in critical care medicine are making it more likely that people will survive serious brain injury. Thus, the actual number of survivors is increasing. Furthermore, as a result of improvements in medicine, the number of survivors with *serious* brain injury is increasing. People are now surviving brain injuries that would once have been fatal but are often left with very serious disabilities.

In summary, in North America we are facing an epidemic of brain injuries that is bringing enormous personal costs to survivors and their families as well as to society. These costs are not only for care and rehabilitation but also in lost work productivity, burden to families, and general misery.

Types of Injuries

Brain injuries are often classified according to severity, as mild, moderate, or severe. Two estimates of severity are the *Glascow Coma Scale (GCS)* and the duration of *post-traumatic amnesia (PTA)*. The *GCS* has three parts: assessment of eye opening, best motor response, and best verbal response. The lowest score is 3, the highest 15. A score of 8 or less is commonly accepted as a 'coma' state and as a *severe brain injury*; a score of 9 to 12 would indicate a *moderate brain injury*; and a score of 13 to 15, a *mild brain injury*. *Post-traumatic amnesia* refers to the time between injury and recovery of continuous memory – that is, full memory for day-to-day events.

A *mild* brain injury can be caused by a motor vehicle accident, a sports incident, a fall, or in fact any event causing a 'bump on the head.' The person would have a GCS score of 13, 14, or 15 and PTA of less than 1 hour. Persons with mild head injuries may receive no medical attention or be hospitalized for observation only. Individuals who suffer a mild head injury, with normal neurological examination results, may experience a wide range of symptoms, including irritability, restlessness, anxiety, and depression. Often, individuals with a mild brain injury are unable to identify what is different about themselves, but know 'something is wrong.' The symptoms and feelings these individuals experience are not apparent to others, as they 'look normal,' and this makes it more difficult for the person with the brain injury to be recognized as having an injury and being in need of proper diagnosis and treatment.

A *moderate* brain injury is characterized by a PTA of 1 to 24 hours and a GCS score from 9 to 12. With a *severe* brain injury the person is in a coma, as determined by a GCS score of 8 or less, that lasts more than one day, and has a PTA of approximately 1 to 7 days. A PTA of over 7 days would indicate a very severe injury.

The Central Nervous System

The brain will be discussed under the following topics: the brain *structure, functions* of the brain, *localization* of brain functions, and *lobes* of the brain.

The Brain Structure   Our brain is what makes us uniquely human. The brain is the organ of the body responsible for what we feel, think, and do. It is responsible for sensations such as vision, hearing, and touch, for voluntary actions such as speaking and walking, for feelings and emotions such as anger and pleasure, for memories, and for decision making or executive functions such as attention, planning, judgment, and being able to correct behaviour.

How does the brain do all this? While we do not have a complete understanding of how the brain works, we do know a considerable amount, and learn more every day. An enormous amount of research is being carried out to improve our understanding of the brain. In the past two decades, new technologies such as imaging techniques have led to major advances in our understanding of brain function.

Like all organs in the body, the brain is composed of billions of microscopic cells. Brain tissue is composed of *nerve cells* or *neurons* and supporting cells known as *glial cells.*

However, *nerve cells* or *neurons* are different from other cells in the body in that they are able to generate pulses of electricity when properly stimulated. These pulses may be transmitted from one neuron to another, or they may terminate; which depends on the strength of the stimulation and on the presence or absence of certain chemicals, called *neurotransmitters.* Thus, the brain and the nervous system operate both electrically and chemically. Information is transmitted in the form of pulses of electricity, from neuron to neuron, if the right chemical conditions are in place.

Neurons are not directly connected to one another. A microscopic gap or *synapse* exists between neurons. The synapse is the site of action of the neurotransmitters. Again, if enough of the correct neurotransmitter is present at the synapse, nerve pulses will be transmitted from one neuron to the next.

The nervous system, which includes the brain and the spinal cord, contains both simple and incredibly complex circuits of neurons. For example, if the hand is touched with sufficient pressure, nerve pulses will be generated in neurons in the hand; these will enter the spinal cord in the neck region. If sufficient neurotransmitter is present in the synapses in the spinal cord, a second set of neurons will carry the pulses to a relay area in the middle of the brain. Finally, a third set of neurons will take the message to the *cortex*, or outer layer of the brain, for interpretation as a touch. Thus, a three-neuron circuit is sufficient to carry a touch message from the hand to the brain for interpretation.

Another simple circuit in the brain is known as a reflex *arc*. Let's take a simple example, such as burning your finger on a hot iron. The hot iron will stimulate the neurons in the finger to give off electrical pulses, which will travel from the hand into the spinal cord and then be transmitted to the brain, causing a sensation of pain.

As with the touch example, this circuit involves three neurons. In the meantime, the pulses entering the spinal cord trigger a stream of pulses going from the spinal cord back to the arm muscles, and this causes a reflex jerking of the finger away from the hot iron. This reflex, which involves the spinal cord and not the brain, being a much faster pathway, reduces the likelihood that the finger will be seriously injured.

The spinal cord is responsible for many of the central nervous system's complex activities, such as those involved in using the hands and walking. In other words, the spinal cord does much more than act as a cable of neurons taking messages to and from the brain.

Before we leave neurons, we should note that they are very susceptible to a shortage or lack of oxygen. If deprived of oxygen (*anoxia*), neurons will begin to die after about seven minutes. Thus, anoxia is a major cause of serious injury to the nervous system.

When neurons in the central nervous system, the brain, and spinal cord die, they are not replaced through regeneration. Neurons outside of the central nervous system, such as in the arms and legs, will regenerate after damage. This means that if a sensory nerve is severed in the arm, sensation will be lost but will return as the neuron grows back.

Again, if damage occurs to neurons in the brain, they do not regenerate or grow back, at least in adults. The reasons for this are not fully understood, and major research efforts are presently underway to understand how neurons might be stimulated to regenerate. If neurons in the central nervous system could be persuaded to grow back, this would have major implications for the treatment of persons with brain and spinal cord injury. It might become possible for the brain and spinal cord to heal, albeit with lost function.

Finally, it should be noted that many neurons are surrounded by a fatty sheath known as *myelin*. Myelin is analogous to the insulation around electrical wires; it increases the speed and efficiency with which information is transmitted along neurons. *Myelination,* which is the formation of myelin sheaths around neurons, is an important part of the development of the nervous system and occurs in the early years of development. Diseases that attack and destroy myelin, such as multiple sclerosis, have serious effects on the functioning of the nervous system.

Structure and Functions of the Brain   The brain is responsible for regulating the body's subcortical or basic life functions such as breathing, heart rate, and temperature maintenance, and for controlling drives such as appetite and thirst. Such things are not normally part of our consciousness or under our voluntary control. Some of these functions, such as breathing, *can* be brought under voluntary control. These functions are called subcortical because they involve 'lower level' centres of the brain (relative to the cerebral hemispheres, which are 'higher level').

Cortical or *cerebral* functions reside in the large, wrinkled cerebral hemispheres, which are the most obvious structures of the human brain. The outer lining of the cerebral hemispheres, or *cortex*, has a greyish appearance and is often referred to as 'grey matter.' This outer cortex is responsible for major sensory functions such as vision, hearing, and touch, for perception (that is, our understanding of sensory information, such as being able to perceive depth), and for other intellectual and executive functions including memory, thinking, planning, attention, and control of behaviour.

Localization of Brain Function Some of the brain's functions are localized in certain regions – for example, those responsible for the control of movement and vision. Other functions, such as cognition and thinking, involve large areas of the brain. Some functions are *lateralized*. Thus, language functions are usually located in the left cerebral hemisphere, while other functions, including spatial ones such as map reading, are lateralized to the right cerebral hemisphere.

The effects of a brain injury will depend on the regions of the brain involved and the extent of damage. Is the damage restricted to a specific area or is it widespread? Is the damage cortical or subcortical? Is the damage in the left or right cerebral hemisphere, or both? Does the damage involve areas where functions are localized, such as the areas responsible for voluntary movement?

To better understand the effects of brain injury, let us briefly consider the major regions of the brain and their functions. When we speak of these regions or *lobes*, we are really discussing the regions of the *cerebral hemispheres*, which are the large, grey, wrinkled structures we normally think of as the brain (See Figure 2.1). Covered by the cerebral hemispheres are the structures of the brainstem responsible for heartbeat, breathing, consciousness, and other key life functions. Also covered by the cerebral hemispheres are the complex structures of the *limbic system*, which are important for emotions such as anger.

Lobes of the Brain The *frontal lobe* is located at the front of the brain. An important task of the frontal lobe is to control voluntary movement or motor behaviour. Thus, a motor action such as raising an arm is initiated in the motor area of the frontal lobe. Motor neurons cross to the opposite side of the body, which means that a command to raise the right arm is initiated by the left frontal lobe. Another

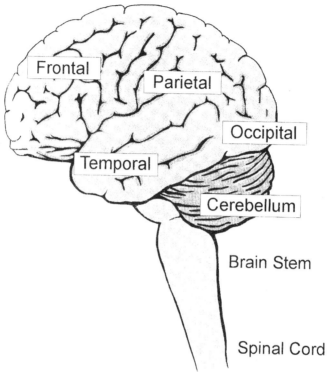

FIGURE 2.1

important function of the frontal lobe is control of speech. As with other language functions, speech in most people is localized in the left hemisphere.

The frontal lobe is also the *executive centre* of the brain, responsible for managing such important human behaviours as planning, paying attention, and making judgments, and for controlling emotions.

All of this means that damage to the frontal lobe can result in the following: involuntary movement or *motor* problems such as weakness or paralysis (involving the opposite side of the body to the injury); difficulties producing speech (referred to as *aphasia* or *dysphasia*); and impairment of executive functions such as paying attention, making judgments, and controlling behaviour.

The actual consequences of the brain injury will depend on which areas of the frontal lobe are involved and the magnitude of the damage. As noted earlier, *how* the damage occurred is not as important as its location and extent.

Because of the effects on the 'executive' or decision-making functions of the brain, damage to the frontal lobe may have especially serious consequences for the survivor and family.

The *temporal lobes* are important for hearing and memory and also for the control of behaviour. These functions are located in *both* temporal lobes. Thus, damage to either the left or the right temporal lobe does not result in major hearing or memory problems. Major deficits will occur only when *both* temporal lobes have been damaged.

We have already discussed how the left cerebral hemisphere is specialized for language. The left temporal lobe is important for the understanding of speech. Damage to the left temporal lobe may result in a deficit where an individual can no longer understand speech.

The *parietal lobe* is a very large lobe of the brain behind the frontal lobe and above the temporal lobe. The parietal lobe is responsible for body sensation – touch, pressure, hot and cold. These body sensations are localized within a relatively thin strip of the parietal lobe. As with motor behaviour, the neurons represent the opposite sides of the body. Thus, the right parietal lobe is responsible for body sensation in the left side of the body.

The parietal lobe is also responsible for a number of complex perceptual functions. Perception is the interpretation by the brain of information reaching it through the sensory systems. Examples of complex perceptual functions in the parietal lobes include recognition of faces and the ability to follow a route such as when driving home. These are examples of functions located in the right parietal lobe.

The left parietal lobe, as might be expected, is important for language related functions. Thus, the brain centre responsible for reading is located in the left parietal lobe.

The *occipital lobes* are responsible for vision. There are quite specific connections between the eyes and the occipital lobes, so damage to a specific area of the occipital lobe in either the left or the right hemisphere will result in a specific blind spot or visual field defect appearing in the left or the right eye. It is important to understand that the eyes do not actually 'see.' Rather, the seeing occurs in the brain. This means that a brain injury involving the occipital lobe will result in a defect in vision. The same applies to the other sensory systems.

Effects of a Brain Injury

Let us now apply this knowledge of the functions of the brain's lobes to explain the effects of brain injuries. For example, what would we expect from a stroke involving the artery that supplies the left frontal lobe? If there was a loss of blood supply to most of the left frontal lobe as a result of this, we would expect paralysis on the *right* side of the body (remember, the nerve fibres cross over), as well as problems in speech (the speech production centre is located in the left frontal lobe).

If there was blockage of the blood supply to the right frontal lobe, the *left* side of the body would be paralysed. However, speech would not be affected, since in most people it is not located in the right frontal lobe.

What would be the effects of a major brain injury involving most of the left hemisphere of the brain? Again, this would result in paralysis and loss of sensation on the right side of the body.

If the damage was extensive enough, there might also be problems in understanding speech and reading. If the damage involved the left occipital lobe, there might be defects in both the left and right visual fields.

If there is extensive damage involving the right hemisphere, paralysis and loss of sensation will occur on the left side of the body. However, there will be no significant impairment of language functions such as speech. Instead, there might be impairment of perceptual functions such as the ability to find the way back to a hospital room, or navigate the way to the kitchen in one's home.

These kinds of problems would be expected with a serious traumatic or nontraumatic brain injury. Again, the *cause* of the injury is not as important as its *location* and *extent*.

Because higher intellectual functions, or those functions which make us uniquely human, are located mainly in the frontal lobe, *fron-*

tal lobe injuries have a special significance. Thus, even a 'mild' frontal lobe injury may have a devastating effect on a survivor and family. Suddenly, that person is no longer the same: there are subtle but significant changes in personality and behaviour. Often these changes make it impossible for the survivor to work in the same job. In many job situations, even small deficits in attention and the ability to plan may cause drastic problems in performance.

The effects on personal relationships are often devastating. The survivor is no longer 'the same person' in a relationship. A frontal lobe injury may lead to serious problems such as impaired judgment and outbursts of aggression. Conversely, the changes in behaviour may be so subtle that they are detected only by partners and close family or friends. These 'subtle' changes may place enormous destructive pressure on partners and family.

Symptoms of a Brain Injury

The symptoms of acquired brain injury are often grouped into these categories:

A. *Cognitive* – involving difficulties in thinking.
B. *Perceptual* – involving problems in interpreting information coming from the senses, such as hearing and vision.
C. *Physical.*
D. *Behavioral and emotional.*

Again, the actual symptoms that appear will depend on the location and extent of the injury, and on the personality of the individual.

A. COGNITIVE SYMPTOMS

- Difficulty in processing information.
- Problems in maintaining attention to tasks
- Impaired decision making.
- Inability to follow a set of instructions.
- Inability to shift attention from one mental task to another.
- Memory loss or impairment.

- Problems in language, such as expressing thoughts or understanding what others are saying.

B. PERCEPTUAL SYMPTOMS

- Changes in vision, hearing, or body sensation such as touch.
- Loss of sense of self, 'who I am.'
- Loss of sense of time.
- Loss of sense of space – where am I and how can I get to somewhere else.
- Disorders of smell.
- Disorders of taste.
- Disorders of balance.
- Changes in pain sensitivity.

C. PHYSICAL SYMPTOMS

- Persistent headache.
- Fatigue.
- Movement disorders – weakness, paralysis, tremors, spasticity, or permanent muscle spasms.
- Epileptic seizures.
- Impairment of fine motor control, such as picking up small objects.
- Sensitivity to light.
- Sleep disorders.
- Speech or articulatory disorders – difficulty pronouncing words.

D. BEHAVIORAL / EMOTIONAL SYMPTOMS

- Irritability.
- Impatience.
- Inability to manage stress.
- Apathy or lack of initiative, lack of energy.
- Dependence on others.
- Denial of disability.

- Lack of inhibition, which may result in aggression, cursing, and inappropriate sexual and other behaviours (such as staring and touching).
- Inability to change behaviour in response to changed circumstances.
- Increased or decreased emotional responding.

Can the Brain Recover from an Injury?

This a difficult question to answer. It depends on the location and extent of the damage and on whether the damage is permanent or temporary. For example, immediately after an accident the brain may swell, resulting in very serious symptoms, which, however, decrease in the ensuing days or weeks. On the other hand, a seemingly 'mild' injury, where there is brief loss of consciousness after a blow to the head, could permanently affect behaviour.

Often, the long-term effects of an injury can be evaluated only after a significant length of time post-injury, and with sophisticated assessment techniques that are sensitive to subtle changes in function and behaviour. Rehabilitation may be effective in restoring functions and reducing the negative long-term effects of brain injury.

In summary, the results of a brain injury are both predictable and to a certain extent unpredictable. What is predictable is that if the injury involves certain structures where functions are located, there will be consequences depending on the location at severity of the injury. Thus, a serious injury to the right frontal lobe will result in a left-sided paralysis.

Unfortunately, what is more difficult to predict is the effect of an injury to the frontal lobes, where the personality and executive functions are located. Damage to this area can be particularly devastating.

3. A Survivor's View

Charles G. Ottewell

I am writing this Journal of my experiences during and after my high school rugby accident in the Spring of 1983. To help myself and to help other people who have suffered a Traumatic Brain Injury or a closed head injury, and to assist family and friends around the brain-injured person, so you can try to understand just what the injured person is trying to cope with in their new world-life.

First I will try to explain what I was like prior to my accident. I was seventeen (17) years old, had a lot of friends, was one of the leaders among my peers. I participated in many sports, from golf and tennis to hockey and skiing. I lifted weights on a regular schedule. In general I was a very motivated and confident person. I was a happy individual and felt like I was in control of my life and had future goals to work toward and to achieve.

The Trauma

It was April 23, 1983, I played rugby for our high school team. I do not have any real memories of that day or playing in that game. People watching the game said I accepted a pass and started running

This chapter was previously published in Ottewell, C.G. (1992). 'From the Patient's Point of View.' *Journal of Cognitive Rehabilitation, 10*(1), 8–12. Reprinted with permission.

with the ball. When I got tackled I took a few more steps before I finally fell down. I then got up, took a few steps, commented about being dizzy, bent over, held my head then collapsed into a coma on the field.

I was then rushed to the local hospital where the medical attendants did as much as they could to keep me alive. My parents were notified of my condition. They rushed to the hospital to see me. It was then decided to fly me to Vancouver in a special Air Ambulance Jet. We had to wait a couple of hours before the plane landed. My mother was permitted to fly with me to Vancouver. Upon arriving at Vancouver, I was then transferred to an ambulance and dispatched to Vancouver General Hospital – V.G.H.

I remained in a coma for a period of up to 3½ weeks. I was kept alive by a number of life-support machines and tubes, each with its own special function – from diagnosing my respiratory problems to my body temperature. I was now breathing through a trachea tube. The heroics of my doctors kept me alive. It was hard for them to believe that it was just a tackle in a rugby game that could cause so much damage. If or when I came out of my coma, they could only guess just how much brain damage I suffered.

While in my coma, I contracted spinal meningitis, which meant another placement of a shunt to my brain to relieve the pressure on my brain. By the third week into my coma, the pressure was still rising and the infection was getting worse. It was decided to pull the shunts off my head and hope I would be around the next morning. It was just another touch-and-go night for me. As the next day was upon us, I was still here. The pressure was beginning to subside on my brain. Finally, of all miracles, I was showing some improvement.

Being in a coma for such a length of time, did destroy my once strong and athletic body. I weighed only 80 pounds, and having no strength or stamina, my personal battle to improve had begun.

Recovery – First Communication

When I came out of my coma, I had no idea where I was or what had happened to me. This is where my mother helped me greatly by showing me pictures and talking to me. I had not much memory loss of things prior to my accident, my family and my friends, but the biggest problem was that my short-term memory was very poor. I could not remember people or events that happened an hour past. My mother would help me by repetition and by questioning me, which did seem to help me improve. I was still unable to communicate, my speech was very slow and slurred. As I got a little bit stronger, I was able to be placed in a wheelchair and buckled in because I did not have enough strength to sit up, and I would slide out. My mother would push me around the endless amounts of hallways discovering new pathways and corridors in the hospital. My major deficits were fairly obvious. I had no real feeling in my legs, the left side of my body was hampered the most. I was unable even to move my fingers or hand. But after a few weeks at V.G.H., a decision was made to transfer me to G.F. Strong Rehabilitation Centre. This move would prove beneficial for me. There was now more outside stimulation and I had to start trying to do more things for myself.

First Memory – Further Recovery

My memory up to this point is very hazy. I really do not have any memory until I was moved to the G.F. Rehabilitation Centre, where I remained for a period of 4 months. I was in a wheelchair for the first 3 months. My trials of being in a wheelchair were very interesting, seeing the world in a different perspective. This was a very confusing period of my recovery. I was first admitted to the 3rd floor and, at this time, I needed a lot of assistance going to the washroom, bathing myself, eating my meals, from dressing myself to tying my own shoes.

My first week at G.F. Strong I was very nervous; my body reacted by hiccupping for about 10 days straight. A very upsetting period of my early recovery. A major problem for me was accepting and admitting my obvious impairments. I did not think I had any. In my mind I thought it was like a broken leg – in a few weeks it would be healed, and everything would be back to normal. At the rehabilitation centre it was a very confusing and difficult time for me. I was not in a familiar setting, and I had to start figuring things out for myself, such as realizing just where I was and just what had happened to me.

Slowly my memory became more clear. Having to interact with more people, having to socialize with other patients and trying to correspond with my doctors and therapists helped. I was now participating in a daily routine of Physiotherapy, cognitive training and gym classes. I was still pushing myself around in my wheelchair, my legs still were not capable of standing or walking. I always knew I was going to walk again, but the big question was when and how well? However, my trials in trying to just push myself around in my wheelchair to eventually standing up, took a very long time and a lot of *tears of strain*. Another problem I had was that I had lost the use of the left side of my body, my leg and arm.

Implications of My Accident

At the centre, I was tested and re-tested regularly. My major deficit physically was not being able to walk, due to the loss of the use of my left side as well as weakness in my right side. Talking was a real chore for me, and my short-term memory was far below normal. The first couple of weeks or so, I had to wear diapers to bed at night. Another problem I encountered as time progressed, was ataxia in the right and left extremities of my body (ataxia is the inability to co-ordinate muscle movements). This hindered my ability to write and even to eat my meals efficiently. My left eye was weakened, with resulting double vision.

So you can see I did not have too many positive things going in my favour. As time went on, even after I left the centre, I still had a lot of *frustrations* and a low-tolerance level, even though I could not see this or admit to it. But this, too, has greatly improved as I have had to learn how to handle certain situations differently and to adjust and cope with them. The key words are *trying* to *accept my new life*. This so-called new me.

Second-stage Recovery: 'Accepting'

Now near the end of the month of July, I was showing some modest improvement. I was able to push myself to the centre's patient cafeteria for my meals, and was able to get in and out of my wheelchair and bed without assistance. However, I still could not change myself, but was able to put on my shoes with limited help.

Meanwhile, I was still at the centre going through my daily routine of physio and gym classes. I had also begun going to school at the centre to see where I was in my education, and to determine how much I was able to manage and comprehend. My speech had improved, but was still very slow and awkward. I was still trying to contend with myself, attempting to accept just where I was and understand my *limitations*. I was experiencing a lot of emotions during this period. As things were becoming more apparent to me, I was slowly realizing that something really did happen to me and my life had changed. I had to relearn practically everything I did, from talking to eating my meals.

I can still recall the huge sense of *loneliness* I felt; it seemed like nobody understood what I was going through. I was the only one, struggling to try and gain back my *independence* and some sort of *normality*. It was a very confusing period of my recovery. Nothing was the same; I had to try and forget who I once was, and learn to live as I am now. But this part of my recovery took a few years more to overcome. It was impossible for me to accept that something really did happen, that I was not going to wake up one morning and everything would be back to normal. I now started fighting heavy bouts of *depression*. I was uncertain where I was and how well I was doing or just what my future had in store for me. I know I did not want to live like I was. I wanted to die; I could not handle the not knowing what I was going to do. I became more angry, had a very low self-esteem and was feeling lost. I experienced grief reaction, admitting that I was *different* now. I had to dramatically change my goals. I had to start life all over again, from stage one, learning to live with myself. I was scared every day of my life, doubtful that I could improve enough physically and mentally to continue living with myself. Everything I tried to do took so long and I could not understand why. Inside my body and brain I thought I was the same person. It was hard for me to believe that there was something wrong with me, that I was not going to get up and walk away.

The wheelchair became an interesting obstacle for me and my parents. We would go to see movies at theatres on the weekends. This caused some problems; we would have to phone ahead to see if the theatre was wheelchair accessible. At one particular theatre there was an escalator going down to the movie. It was a tight squeeze, but my chair just fitted in. The usher then roped off the entrance and took me down with no difficulty. After the movie was over, the usher once again squeezed my chair into the escalator for the ride to the top. But he forgot to rope off the crowd of people behind us. All went well until we reached the top, where my wheelchair got jammed in the narrow opening of the escalator. But the escalator did not stop, and people kept piling on behind my wheelchair, with no place to go. Eventually something had to give, finally the pressure of people forced my wheelchair to pop out just like a cork in a bottle of champagne, and I rolled free. It was one of the lighter sides of being in a wheelchair.

Encouragement

One of my biggest days at the centre was during physiotherapy class. We would have to lock the brakes on our wheelchairs, and the physiotherapist would time us and see how long we could stand up before collapsing onto the mat on the floor. This particular day, I stood up for an amazing 23 seconds, my therapist screamed and we just about had a party. Finally I saw some sort of real improvement. My legs finally worked, although not for very long, but it did give some much needed *encouragement* to keep pushing myself. This accelerated my progress in gym class.

It was now August, four months since my injury, and I persevered. I now could actually stand up and take a couple of steps between the parallel bars with assistance from my gym teacher, who had to help me move my legs so I could continue to walk. Gym class was my favourite class, as it was here that I was able to push myself more physically and see some sort of improvement.

Continued Progress

As far as my school work went, I was far below my grade expectations. This was also a very *trying* time for me because physically it was almost impossible for me to even hold a pen or pencil, as the ataxia in my hands was so bad. But I kept forcing myself to think, and with the aid of writing apparatus, my writing did improve, until at least I could use a normal size pen. Once again my major goal by attending school at the centre was to improve enough so I could return home and continue my education at my own school. My reading was hindered by double vision. With reading and writing skills being so poor, my ambition to continue on with school was a lot further away than I presumed. It seemed like I was always setting such unrealistic goals for myself. But this particular goal of going back home, continuing my education and graduating from Grade 12 with my class, was more than enough *motivation* to keep me struggling with the tedious task at hand. Still in August, I was getting quite desperate, knowing summer holidays were just about over, and school was about to start again. I knew I had to return home soon if I wanted to try and graduate with my class.

I was still quite uncertain of what had happened to me. Nothing in my life was the same. In a sense, I was still trying to figure out what I was really capable of doing. I always thought I should accomplish more than I was able to, which left me mentally discouraged and depressed.

You could say that I was not the happiest individual you have ever met. Which meant being around me could be very tiring for my family. I am sure my parents had to develop a pretty thick skin, so to speak, to deal with my negative attitude, which lasted for at least up to a year after my accident. I was still learning how to act socially acceptable in certain situations.

As the month of September approached, my physical rehabilitation kept progressing quite well. I was now able to walk by pushing my wheelchair. I still used my wheelchair when I got too tired of standing up. My schooling was slowly improving, but still far below grade expectancy, but I was determined to return home and try to graduate with my class at school. I could not 'accept' being left behind a year and continuing my education a year later, not unless I gave it a good honest effort, to see if I could do it.

I think the physical part was attainable, but the big question was intellectual. Was I ready and able to 'accept' the responsibility that I would encounter when I did return home to continue my studies? I was becoming more and more *stubborn*. I wanted to return home so much! I felt my progress at the centre was limited. I was not going to be 'able' to improve enough or fast enough if I remained at the centre.

The entire staff at the centre, from the orderlies to my physiotherapist and gym therapist, were all very supportive and very helpful in rehabilitating me to my fullest potential. The centre's doctors and directors showed a lot of empathy for me, and I am sure they wanted whatever was best for me, to stay at the centre or to return home.

As the month of October approached, I think I knew it was now or never if I had a chance to return home and continue on with my *life*. My improvement with my attitude had begun to slow down. My therapists were becoming more unaware of what to do for me. I was becoming more depressed and anxious. Soon it was decided to have my annual team meeting, with all my doctors, psychologist, therapist and parents. It was decided it would be more beneficial for me to try and return to home and school. At last my dream to return home came true. I was elated and felt like I could conquer anything in my path now. I had improved enough so that I was able to be discharged and go home.

The Return Home

I thought returning home would answer all my questions and self-doubts. But when I did arrive home, I did not realize that I had changed as a person. The most obvious change was my physical appearance, walking with a cane. And I was still trying to live with myself, trying to cope with this so-called new me. I did at first have some social problems, doing and saying things at inappropriate times. A lot of my friends did not talk or even try to socialize with me. I found out in a hurry, just who were my *real friends*. I realize now it was their maturity level. I appreciate those individuals so much for at least trying to understand and sticking beside me. This part of my recovery also took awhile to overcome. To myself, I felt like the same person, liked doing the same things as before my accident, although I was unable to do a lot of things. I always thought I would wake up one morning and everything would be back to normal. It was like a bad dream, this was not really happening to me. This, too, took some time to adjust to.

School was unbearable. I could not have imagined it being so tough. In a sense I was still re-learning, re-teaching myself how to read and write, and retraining my memory. I was becoming more and more depressed. Most of my teachers were supportive, and I did get a tutor who would help me read and write out my assignments, which was a great asset for me to keep up with my classes at school. I also needed a lot of counselling support, in which I am truly grateful that a certain counsellor was there for me. With my frustration and depression getting worse, that counsellor listened and helped me through a lot of dark periods that last year of school.

One of the hardest things that I can recall, was feeling like the *only one*. I thought everybody was staring at me, yet I felt like the old me, before my accident. I tried to go out on the weekends but felt 'awkward.' So, I spent a lot of time by *myself*. I liked being *alone* with my own thoughts, realizing just where I was.

My parents were very supportive, they knew that my goal was to graduate with my class. They did their best to keep me 'active' in doing my school work. I can only imagine what they must have been going through. My *anger*, a lot of the time, was focused on them. I am not sure exactly why. I was trying so hard and getting no acceptable results for myself, and did not like them seeing me struggling and, a lot of the time, failing. I was becoming somewhat more uncontrollable, swearing and lashing out, trying to hide my *insecurities*. My parents had to develop a lot of tolerance and try to live with me during this part of my recovery. Just about every day, I would have an emotional break-down of some sort after I arrived home from school.

I attempted to work out with the set of weights that I had at home, always thinking that I could regain everything that I had lost. My father would help me. I used to try and run up and down our driveway. My dad would help me by moving my left arm accordingly with the right side of my body. I used to get so angry at myself when I could not succeed at something like trying to run. This part of my physical ability still eludes me today, but I still have not completely given up my dream to be able to run one block or even just ten feet.

Another problem I had in working out was that my energy level was low after going to school every day and doing homework. So, I stopped exercising and tried just to cope with my schooling. I did have to do a lot of walking at school, so I was still getting some exercise. It was like I was on *a mini rollercoaster ride*; some *ups* and definitely a lot of *downs*. Life was getting so hard; some days seemed to last forever. My confusion with myself was still very apparent. I went to see a psychologist who specialized with patients who had injuries similar to mine. He did a number of tests on me to see where I was intellectually, what and how much I was capable of doing in school, what kinds of learning assistance would be most beneficial for me. The results of these tests showed some strong and weak areas, but still, far below the level of grade 12. My ambition to finish school that year was becoming more unlikely, a fact which I could not accept. So, I continued on with my daily routine.

Everything in my life, from tying my shoes, to reading a book was a laborious affair. Some mornings when I woke up the left side of my body did not work, I could barely walk, my left arm and hand became totally useless to me. But, I 'forced' myself to take my morning shower, get dressed, have breakfast and get ready to go to school. I tried to make my left hand do as much as it could. I had to carry my books in my left arm at school, for I had to use my walking cane in my right hand. When I had enough time, I made my left hand open and close my locker door at school to retrieve what books I needed for my next class. At times, this process, which should only take a couple of seconds, took a few minutes; trying to coordinate my hand to do what I was telling it to do.

My writing was still very much hampered by my ongoing fight with ataxia in my hand. So, at the end of every day, my concentration in doing just everyday tasks, would leave me more than just a little bit exhausted. But I did not let on just how much trouble I was having. I was trying to show that I was as independent as I ever was and in control of my actions and my life.

I passed my courses in the first semester, and this gave me some much needed motivation to continue on with my classes for the second semester. The last month of school, I was still struggling with my classes, and still was only dreaming of graduating that year. I had to start studying for my final exams. This is where my defeatist attitude negatively affected my fragile confidence. I would not study as hard as I knew I should for I did not have the confidence in myself and my memory to pass an exam. I was convinced that I would fail.

As the last couple of weeks of school drew nearer, I was still passing my courses. I still spent a lot of free time by myself, almost as if I was a *social outcast* to the rest of my graduating class. Finally, the longest school year that I could have imagined came to an end. My dream and struggle to graduate with my peers came true. When I received my certificate that graduation ceremony, I received a *standing applause from the audience*. I was elated and so happy for my family and parents, I *proved* to myself and them that I could do it. It was the first time in at least a year that I truly felt good and positive about myself.

Summer holidays finally came. I had to start thinking of what I was going to do in the future. I wanted to start exercising, so I could get back into shape and be able to look after myself more independently. I worked hard to try and improve myself physically by working out and doing physiotherapy. But, I would get very little positive results, which still today eludes me. I am not sure if it will ever be possible for me to improve my strength, stamina and co-ordination to how I once was. I just have to keep persisting, so at least I should not get any worse. This is also a *most frustrating* fact of *reality* I have to admit to, and have to accept and live with.

Summer came to an end and I was still living at home. I took a trip by myself to Vancouver to check out some post secondary schools and colleges. This minor trip proved beneficial for me, allowing me to push myself physically and mentally and gain a sense of independence. It was my own motivation and responsibility that I took upon myself to head back to school.

Independence

So the move was on, I signed up for a couple of courses at a community college that Spring Semester. The counsellors I met with were very understanding and supportive. They had learning assistance, such as tutors who could assist me with my reading and writing. My first semester was a growing experience. With the counsellor's help I ended up taking a single course which did occupy all my time. I soon realized that I was not capable of doing a full course load, so I did as much as I could. Living independently, paying a monthly rent, and cooking my own meals made me feel like I was getting some control over my life. It was easier meeting new people and friends because they saw me as I am now and could relate to me easier. This is the real me, walking with a slow gait and a walking cane. I did not have to try and be something that I am not, which I think was one of my *major problems* back at home in that last year of school. I was learning to accept myself, and hoping others could accept me as I was as well.

Another distressing problem that I have encountered is that I have not been able to sleep well since the accident. Insomnia at its worse, which is getting harder to live with, not being able to relax and rest. This does not make my schooling and studying any easier. What I understand is that this can be a problem for many traumatic brain injured survivors. My major problem is I am unable to shut off my brain, so I am always thinking of what I did today, what I am going to do tomorrow. So this is hampering a lot of my abilities to study more efficiently and have enough energy to exercise more effectively. Still, being at school, plugging away at one or two courses a semester, and being able to care and depend on myself is a *major accomplishment* for me.

I was still somewhat depressed because I wanted to do more, but I was still unable to do so. My sleeping was getting worse, I had such a high stress level, which I still do today. I still wonder why? And how? I am managing my affairs, I look at every day as a *new fight*.

Conclusion

With traumatic brain injuries, there are no two exact same brain injuries. Everyone who has suffered one is unique. But, there are a lot of parallels between them, be it the denial that anything really did happen to you, or the anger of trying to understand what has happened to you. The darkest fact is the obvious *depression* one has to live through which I don't know will ever end. I think the depression becomes less, and definitely not as strong, for I am still here, fighting to make a life for myself, and I do not want to end my life. All I can say is that I think the injured person has to be given a fair chance, and set some sort of goals for themselves, from being able to tie one's shoes, to making a phone call by themselves. These small achievements, which are huge to the individual, will give them some much needed confidence to try and gain some sort of independence. One of the biggest assets I think I had, and which I believe propelled me to keep moving forward, was my *motivation*. It was so strong, to attempt to graduate with my class, and gain back some *independence* and normality. I think you have to have some sort of motivation, whatever it may be. Another most important factor is to be able to succeed at a certain task. I now realize how important it was for me to prevail at first, just being able to put on my own shoes without assistance, to eventually standing up and actually taking a step.

I thank the staff and doctors at G.F. Strong Rehabilitation Centre for having the insight to let me try. I appreciate the tremendous support and understanding that I received from my parents, who a lot of the time were my *backbone*.

I have climbed a lot of mountains, and there always seems to be another mountain for me to challenge. I was not supposed to live. If I did, I would do so as a 'human vegetable.' I suppose I am lucky, if I dare use that word, that I lived and can remember living in both worlds, as a normal person and now as a brain injured person. So, I've lived on both sides of the fence, and I am now straddling on either side. I had to, and still am, fighting life everyday. Life is very frustrating and hard for me. I am still bitter and angry. I have accomplished more than anyone could have imagined. But I still have a lot more achievements to accomplish before I can say I have truly won this fight. This accident has altered my life negatively in every way. I had to grow up and mature very quickly, to adjust to myself and how I was thinking. So, I hope other traumatic brain injured individuals have as much support as I did, and are *stubborn* enough to try pushing themselves as hard as it takes. Family and friends need to try to understand and be very patient with the individual. Things may not seem to improve weekly or monthly, but if you are encouraged to keep trying, you will notice many improvements. Years later you will learn how to cope with different situations. I will admit I fell down lots, but always managed to pick myself up and continue on. Things will improve, although not as well or as quickly as you would like. But you did survive from your predicament, so I hope brain-injured individuals are *counselled* to know what their capabilities and responsibilities can be. Every day is a *fight*, from carrying a half a cup of coffee to the kitchen table, to reading a novel or a textbook. So, I hope one day I will *truly* become at *peace* with *myself*, and I hope other brain injured individuals are given a *chance* to show what they are really capable of providing to the society in which they reside.

4. After the Brain Injury – The Rehabilitation Team

John Higenbottam, PhD

Damage Control

When a brain injury occurs, the immediate priority is damage control. This is the *acute* phase of treatment and takes place in hospital. Persons with serious brain injuries may require critical care, including life support for vital functions – breathing, nutrition, and excretion of wastes. Drug therapies are used to control infection and to minimize cell damage and swelling of the brain. If the brain injury is due to stroke or bleeding within the skull, steps are taken to stop the bleeding and relieve the pressure to the brain.

The clinical professionals or *disciplines* involved in the acute phase are mainly physicians and nurses. Among the physicians involved in the acute phase are neurologists and neurosurgeons. *Neurology* is concerned with diseases and damage to the nervous system; *neurosurgery* involves specialized surgical procedures involving the brain, the spinal cord, and other nerves in the body. Removing a tumour, for example, is a neurosurgical procedure.

Once the survivor's medical condition has been stabilized, the focus switches to rehabilitation.

Members of the Rehabilitation Team

In this chapter we will focus on the members of the rehabilitation team and their responsibilities in assessing and rehabilitating the

Physiatrist	Physiotherapists
Nurses	Recreational therapists
Clinical psychologist	Dietitian
Neuropsychologist	Vocational rehabilitation specialists
Psychiatrist	Teachers
Social worker	Sexual health clinician
Speech/language pathologists	Chaplain
Occupational therapists	

FIGURE 4.1 Members of the Rehabilitation Team

brain-injured survivor (see Figure 4.1 for a listing of team members). The therapies used by these professionals are also described. Depending on the injury sustained and the facility the survivor is in, some or all of the members of the rehabilitation team may be involved. It is critical that the survivor and the family, as well as the case manager (if one has been identified), be involved in team discussions and decisions.

Physiatrists are physicians who specialize in rehabilitation medicine. They are often the leaders of the rehabilitation team, and are responsible for assessing the client's needs and drawing up the rehabilitation plan. The physiatrist is often the main point of contact among the rehabilitation team – the person to whom physicians, the family, and lawyers and insurers are referred.

Nurses are responsible for providing twenty-four-hour care throughout hospital rehabilitation. Accordingly, they provide most of the care that a patient receives in a rehabilitation unit. They work closely with other clinicians to provide care in the areas of physical, cognitive, and emotional functioning. Nurses are a major source of information for survivors and families as rehabilitation proceeds.

Clinical psychologists are experts in behaviour. Psychologists are involved in dealing with the emotional and behavioural issues that often arise after brain injury. In dealing with these issues, psychologists will involve family members and caregivers.

Neuropsychologists are clinical psychologists who specialize in the brain injury and behaviour. They conduct assessments to identify cognitive deficits or problems in thinking, memory, and perception; they also track the changes in behaviour that may accompany a brain injury.

When deficits and problems are identified, the neuropsychologist works with the other members of the rehabilitation team to develop a rehabilitation program intended to restore or compensate for cognitive deficits. Restoring cognitive functions is often referred to as *cognitive retraining* or *rehabilitation*.

Dealing with behavioural and emotional issues may involve counselling and psychotherapy as well as the use of medications. If medications are required to deal with problems in behaviour, these will often be prescribed by a *psychiatrist*, who is a physician specializing in the management of abnormal behaviour and emotional problems.

Social workers may also provide counselling and psychotherapy to survivors and their families. They are also responsible for arranging social service benefits and for exploring appropriate community living arrangements when it is time for the survivor to leave the hospital.

Speech/language pathologists are clinical specialists who deal with problems of speech, language, and communication associated with a brain injury. As discussed in chapter 2, injuries involving the left hemisphere may result in speech and language deficits – for example, the inability to produce or understand speech. Speech/language therapy focuses on assessing these language disorders and retraining the individual. In some situations, where the individual has lost completely the ability to speak, an alternative communication system may be required, such as a symbol or computer board that allows the survivor to spell out messages.

Damage to the brain stem may result in problems with swallowing, which can be a discomfort and possibly hazardous to the survivor. The mechanisms of swallowing are very complex, and treatment often involves several disciplines, including speech/language pathologists and dietitians or nutritionists. Sophisticated fluoroscopic techniques are often needed to evaluate and treat swallowing problems. Fluoroscopy is a type of X-ray technique that allows the actual process of swallowing to be observed and analysed.

Occupational therapists are key rehabilitation professionals who help the brain injury survivor restore function and develop living skills to deal with his or her deficits. The aim of occupational therapy is to train clients in skills such as personal hygiene, money management, shopping, and meal preparation. The goal here is to allow clients to function in the community with the greatest possible independence. When certain skills cannot be developed because of the results of the injury, the focus of the therapy must change: to help the survivor learn techniques that will compensate for lost abilities. In other words, the individual is taught to do things in a *different* way to deal with his or her deficit. For example, the use of a memory journal can help compensate for memory loss. The survivor can use the journal to plan daily activities, with the entries serving as prompts to carry out certain activities at certain times of day. A journal also helps survivors recall events. The survivor may need assistance with making the journal entries, depending on his or her abilities.

Physiotherapists are specialists in body movement, or *motor functions*. Through a structured physiotherapy program, the physiotherapist attempts to restore normal muscle functioning such as that involved in using the hands, or walking. If normal functioning cannot be restored, approaches are taught that help compensate for the deficit. For example, in the case of an activity such as walking, the individual might be taught to use an assistive device such as a cane. If the survivor is actually in a coma, the physiotherapist, in conjunction with other members of the rehabilitation team, may use a therapy called *coma stimulation*. Sound, light, and physical touch are used to assist in recovery from coma (which is defined as a prolonged loss of or reduction in consciousness).

Recreation therapists specialize in restoring leisure and recreational abilities. Leisure and recreational activities are among the most important parts of anyone's life, and a critical area in rehabilitation; these activities are discussed in more detail in chapter 14.

Dietitians advise on proper nutrition, which is critical in promoting recovery and healthy living. Dietitians play a key role in counselling clients and family in the hospital and after return to community living.

Vocational rehabilitation specialists are concerned with maximizing the potential of the brain-injured client to return to meaningful work, which is an enormously important part of any person's life. Vocational assessment and planning are key aspects of the rehabilitation process. Where necessary, 'voc/rehab' specialists will arrange additional training and educational opportunities to help survivors achieve vocational goals.

Other clinical disciplines may well play an important part in the client's rehabilitation, depending on the nature of the problems present after the brain injury. With younger clients, for example, *teachers* play a key role in academic planning and re-entry into the educational system. Also, teachers may provide adult basic education to older survivors, if this is important to their rehabilitation.

Sexual health clinicians are specialists in sexual functioning. Sexuality is an important area of life. If there are disturbances of sexual functioning associated with the brain injury, it is important to involve sexual health clinicians with the survivor and family.

The *chaplain* attends to the spiritual needs of individuals and is a key individual in rehabilitation working with the client, other members of the rehabilitation team, and the family.

Assessing Care Needs

Throughout the recovery period, various members of the health disciplines will contribute to the assessment of the needs of the survivor. In the acute phase, the focus is on medical and nursing investigations, with other specialized clinical practitioners involved as required. In rehabilitation, the physiatrist psychologists, and social workers play a more predominant role. Let's look at some of the assessments done at various stages of recovery.

In acute care, the *neurological examination* provides the most important information for planning treatment. By assessing a client's sensory, motor, and cognitive functioning, the neurological examination identifies significant brain damage or dysfunction.

Other assessment information is important, to add to the basic information gained through the neurological examination. *Electroencephalography* (EEG) has been used for many years to identify areas of the brain that are damaged or are not functioning normally. The EEG measures the electrical activity of the brain's neurons and can identify areas of abnormality fairly precisely. In recent years, computers have been coupled with EEGs to identify areas of abnormality that are difficult to identify through traditional EEG procedures.

Other technologies that have been developed in the past twenty years are contributing greatly to our understanding of brain function and to our ability to evaluate brain damage or dysfunction. These new technologies are known as *imaging* technologies, because they allow us to 'see' brain structures without opening the skull. *Computerized axial tomography*, often referred to as *CAT scanning*, is a technology based on computer enhancement of skull X-rays. This technique can provide detailed images of brain structures and identify damaged areas.

Magnetic resonance imaging (MRI), another new imaging technology, generates very clear and detailed images of brain structure using the energy given off by brain neurons. MRI can provide incredibly detailed images to help identify areas of brain injury.

A third imaging technique, *positron emission tomography (PET)*, is capable of evaluating the metabolic functioning of brain tissue. Metabolic functioning refers to the ability of tissue to use food and oxygen. The PET scan identifies regions of the brain that have abnormally high or low activity. With stroke, for example, the blood supply to a region of the brain will be reduced, thereby reducing its metabolic activity. This reduced activity is clearly visible with a PET scan.

These developments in imaging technology have contributed sub-stantially to improved care and treatment of persons with brain injury.

In the *rehabilitation hospital*, other types of clinical assessment become important, and each member of the care and rehabilitation team contributes to the assessment with the goal of planning and providing the most appropriate treatment. A *neuropsychological assessment* is necessary to evaluate deficits in cognitive functions, and in higher intellectual functions such as attention, perception, and memory. Speech/language pathologists carry out evaluations of speech and verbal functioning. Occupational therapists and physio-therapists evaluate sensory, motor, and cognitive functions as well.

From the information provided by these practitioners, an inter-disciplinary treatment plan is developed for the client. This plan includes long-term goals for the client, as well as specific short-term objectives ('short-term' in the sense of the next weeks or months). These goals and objectives are set by the team with the input and agreement of the client and family. The client, family, and team can then evaluate the client's progress toward the objectives and goals.

This *interdisciplinary approach* to the client reflects an understand-ing that no single discipline can meet all the client's needs. This awareness is at the core of effective rehabilitation. Most clients have a multitude of rehabilitation needs, and only through an effective interdisciplinary approach can these needs be evaluated and addressed. Most importantly, this interdisciplinary process *should involve the client (survivor) and family.* For rehabilitation to be effec-tive, it must involve a partnership of specialists, clients, and family.

5. The Hospital – and After

Rick Brown, MSW, RSW

The day has finally arrived. The brain-injured survivor is at yet another turning point in the long journey called 'recovering from a brain injury' – the survivor is finally leaving the hospital. This event will most likely be a continuation of the emotional roller-coaster ride that began with the accident. Survivors may be experiencing mixed feelings about discharge – feelings ranging from happiness to fear, from anxiety to depression.

On the one hand, survivors may feel as though it is all over: they have made it through the toughest part and things will now return to normal because they are going home. Others may feel that they have no control over their lives. Family members are often worried about their ability to provide care for the injured survivor, who so far has been nurtured by a small army of health care professionals. At this point in time, the survivor will be experiencing many different feelings, not one of which is 'wrong.' Recovery is affected by a number of things, including the nature and severity of the injury, the length of coma, posttraumatic amnesia, the quality of emergency and acute care treatment, pre-injury personality, availability of needed rehabilitation services, and the support of family and friends.

For everyone involved, the client's leaving the hospital and getting prepared for the next stage of recovery is a challenging experience. As a social worker in an acute care rehabilitation hospital, my work with many caregivers, family members, and brain injury survivors has helped me understand how the survivor feels during this time. Perhaps the most important lesson I've learned is that each brain injury survivor is *unique*, and so is his or her family. Every person deals with the recovery from a brain injury using different strategies and at a different speed. This means that I cannot provide here a specific and straightforward plan for coping with discharge from hospital. I *can*, however, raise a number of issues to be considered, which I hope will serve as a guide through the often confusing and uncertain recovery process.

The Rehabilitation Phase

Just when survivors are beginning to recognize and understand the health care team in the acute care hospital, they are discharged to the rehabilitation facility, where they encounter a whole new team, known as the *rehabilitation team* (the roles of the different team members were described in chapter 4). The family, partner, and close friends are also a team. Within this family team, someone must serve as a leader. The family team leader must be flexible, adaptable, and capable of being different things to different people. At all times, the family team leader maintains close communication with the professional team, and serves as the link between the two teams.

By this point in their recovery, the brain injury survivors themselves may be able to identify the best candidate for family team leader. Some survivors, like injured players, may recognize that for a period of time their contributions to the team will necessarily be less than optimal.

A clearly defined family team leader, or better yet, two team leaders, should be designated, even if only on a temporary basis. The leader(s) will 'call the plays' and, it is hoped, be supported by the rest of the family team. Controversy may sometimes arise over the leadership; certain family members may assert that they would do the job better, or become convinced that their methods are the only way. This can create an additional source of stress for all concerned. It is important that everyone involved make an effort to put differences aside and work in the best interests of the survivor. Depending on the time available to family members and their knowledge of the often complex array of formal programs, there may be a need for a case manager – for someone who is knowledgable about the health care system and other systems the survivor will be in contact with (see chapter 6 for information on case management).

While in rehabilitation care, the survivor and family may hear reference to another scale, called the *Rancho Los Amigos Scale (RLA)*, which is often used for assessing the progress of the survivor during recovery. The RLA scale, developed by the brain injury treatment team at Rancho Los Amigos Hospital in California, has eight levels of progressive response and state of awareness. These flow from Level 1, where there is no response (the person is in a coma), through to Level 8, where the individual is alert and essentially independent. If you hear reference made to the use of the RLA scale in the care of your family member, ask for a copy of the scale and an explanation of the different levels of alertness.

Residential Care or Home?

Discharge from the acute rehabilitation hospital may be to one's own home or to a residential facility. The following are some important issues to consider in making the decision: type and severity of injury; finances; types and location of residential facilities; family role changes; educational and vocational issues; transportation needs; daily routines; need for supervision; visitors' requirements; communication with the rehabilitation team; legal, avocational, and social support; and spiritual and caregiver needs. Some of these will be discussed here, others in later chapters.

Finances are often disrupted when a family member sustains a brain injury, and compensation is usually based on how the injury occurred. If the injury was incurred on the job, the survivor may be eligible for Workers' Compensation. If a motor vehicle was involved, litigation may follow. Alternatively, the survivor may be eligible for wage indemnities, or for rehabilitation funding from an insurance company, or for federal, provincial, or state disability insurance. Financial matters are important and need to be thoroughly reviewed following a brain injury. The case manager or a health care professional can direct you to a knowledgeable person in this area.

Survivors may need to request a leave of absence from their employer. This, however, requires that the appropriate forms be completed, which in turn may require supporting medical documentation. Survivors need a capable and persistent advocate to represent them through this process. The case manager can assist here; if there isn't one, it is best to consult a social worker or lawyer. Uncertainties and time delays are the norm with respect to financial matters. This is the time when survivors are in greatest need of financial support, yet ironically, this is also when all the 'fine print' of contracts suddenly becomes real. As a result, time delays are common. Each situation is different, as is the response of each financial agency.

In terms of *residential placement*, this again depends on the type and severity of the brain injury, and on what community resources are available. Residential options include the following: return home; relocation from the previous residence to one adapted to the survivor's needs; longer-term rehabilitation in another facility; or a group home with other brain-injured survivors.

Any decision brings with it additional considerations. If the survivor goes home, adaptations to the physical layout may be necessary. It is best if these modifications are made prior to discharge. Issues to be considered include these: 'Does the survivor require in-home support?' 'Can the family provide any supervision?' 'Do family members have to change their routines to accommodate the needs of the survivor?' 'What resources are available, and who can I talk to about this?'

Regarding *family role changes*, power struggles sometimes develop within the family, especially between family caregivers and the survivor. For good reason, the caregivers have become protective of the brain injury survivor. Conversely, the brain injury survivor may be at a stage where he or she is appropriately trying to regain some sense of independence and control. A classic scenario is that of a brain-injured husband returning home with a desire to drive the family car, despite the rehabilitation team's advice to the contrary. If the wife attempts to intervene, the husband may respond with anger, seeing this as some form of conspiracy against his attempts to regain some independence. This puts the wife in an awkward situation, and it can become stressful for both parties: perhaps the wife was not used to challenging her husband's judgment prior to his injury. This illustrates only one of the many possible role changes within the family. Another example: the wife, who is the injured party, had previously managed the family finances; the husband must now assume these responsibilities. Learning new roles is not easy for anyone.

Whether the injury to the brain is mild, moderate, or severe, the brain-injured survivor's abilities change. This can be very distressing to others, as the survivor may not have total insight into his or her situation. The coping strategies that brain injury survivors develop during the rehabilitation phase of recovery often include these: denial that they have any problems, anger about their situation, depression, hostility, aggression, suicidal thoughts, lack of interest in day-to-day activities, an unusual degree of relaxation, the need for frequent sleep (or altered sleep patterns), the development of a reliance on alcohol or illicit drugs, and extreme dependence on others. Family members should try to be aware of these reactions.

Children in the home can encounter problems, whether they are infants, toddlers, adolescents, or adults. Former ways of relating to the brain injury survivor may no longer work. How will family members deal with, and feel about, these changes? Let's not forget about extended family, neighbours, acquaintances, colleagues, and so on. Do they understand the effects of brain injury? What kind of information do they really need, or want? Do the survivors themselves have enough information to contend with this? Are they comfortable talking about the injury? Will the brain-injured survivor be part of these discussions? How will the survivors deal with comments like these? 'He/she/you look(s) fine.' 'Seems exactly the same as they were.' 'A friend of mine had a complete recovery.' or 'Don't worry, he/she/you is/are lucky to be alive'?

How do survivors regain control over their lives? People are creatures of habit. By this point, family and friends have probably established new routines that differ radically from those prior to the injury. This is a time to review and reflect on these changes. Survivors may need to re-establish a few of their former routines before all of the new changes become too established.

Initially, many family caregivers believe they must focus exclusively on the needs of the brain injury survivor. In time, however, they may find it impossible to continue along this path without taking time out for themselves, to 'recharge.' Earlier on, caregivers may not know what they will need. It's common for others to offer assistance, as in, 'If you need any help, just let us know.' Typically, the caregivers are uncomfortable, or unable to let others help. It will sometimes emerge that caregivers think it unnecessary to ask for help, as in 'Others should know what I need.' However, most people do not really know how to offer assistance, because they do not know what is appropriate. Caregivers may then believe that the offers of help were not genuine.

Perhaps the best solution is for family caregivers to recognize early on in the recovery process that they need to involve as many other people as possible. Ideally, more than one person will share the responsibilities. Again, the family team leader can 'quarterback' this operation by knowing which plays are required and what others can do to provide support.

The Long Term

Long-term expectations for survivors differ in each situation. Following are some general comments about what to anticipate during the course of recovery:

Recovery from a brain injury is always a slow process. The realistic aim is slow, steady progress. Brain injury survivors need time to work out who they are, and will eventually come to realize that they will forever be different. While this is coming about, they may be unable to appreciate the permanent effects of their condition on others. Caregivers sometimes come to resent what they perceive as selfishness on the survivors' part. Caregivers often feel that there is a lack of recognition for all the contributions and sacrifices they have made. Conversely, brain injury survivors may meet with resistance in their attempts to re-establish their independence. Caregivers are often reluctant to let go, not out of meanness but because they care.

Vocational issues become important. So does any involvement in meaningful, productive activities, which are critical to anyone's sense of self-worth. Socializing is another priority, as is the creation of opportunities to meet new people. New acquaintances may accept the brain injury survivor for who he or she is *now* instead of comparing the survivor with his or her pre-injury self.

In the long term, social isolation can occur if the caregivers, or brain injury survivors, shut themselves off emotionally and physically from others. They may, however, feel that others are withdrawing from them. Friends and relatives are sometimes afraid to initiate conversations with the brain-injured survivor, because they do not know what is appropriate. This is where education and direct communication both become important. A good question to ask others is, 'What do you understand about this brain injury?' Survivors are often surprised at the responses to this question. Whatever the response, it is good to begin at whatever level of understanding others are at. Survivors as educators can help to dispel misconceptions regarding what brain injury is and is not. Support groups and brain injury associations can also help the family and survivor obtain additional information on the long-term effects of brain injury, and attendance at these groups can help prevent feelings of isolation (see chapter 15 for more information on support groups).

In summary, the departure from the hospital and the many events that follow will vary with each given situation. Establishing a family team leader, and engaging a case manager if needed, can ease the recovery process and help the survivors work through their inevitable changes and transitions. It is also important to allow survivors to determine their own recovery pace, and to encourage all parties not to lose sight of their own needs. Everyone needs private time. Recognizing that each person involved will employ a different coping style and deal with matters according to a different timetable will help everyone understand and tolerate differences.

Engaging the support of others is easier when there has been adequate education about what to expect. Keep in mind that the experience is new for everyone. Asking for help and information from health care professionals is important.

Brain-injured survivors will need to establish as much independence as they are capable of. They will need opportunities to find out what they can and cannot do. Family members will be trying to establish new relationships and communication strategies with survivors.

Change does not have to be a negative experience. Adversity some-times brings with it opportunities for growth. With or without a brain injury, life includes risks, challenges, and setbacks. The ability to adapt can create new perspectives and opportunities; it can provide challenges, achievements, and unexpected rewards that enhance the road to recovery.

6. Case Management

John Simpson

We have come to expect that when a member of a family becomes ill or has been injured in some kind of incident, that person will see a doctor. There will be some treatment in an emergency department, a stay in hospital, a course of treatment and/or surgery, and perhaps rehabilitation, after all of which life will return to normal. When there has been a relatively minor injury or an illness, we see our family doctor, who will make the appropriate referrals, again, after a period of time life will return to normal and we will carry on with school or work and with life at home.

As was discussed in earlier chapters, brain damage can be caused in many, many different ways. There can be brain damage from a near-drowning incident; from lack of oxygen to the brain during a severe heart attack; from the removal of a tumour or aneurysm; from a sports injury, regardless of the protective equipment worn; or, of course, from an accident such as a car crash or a fall. After any of these, a family faces a maze of care decisions and a long period of rehabilitation. There will be meetings with doctors on a one-to-one basis or with a team taking care of the injured person. A great deal of information will be offered in a relatively short period of time, much of which may be confusing. With all the stress that accompanies the situation, the family will absorb only a fraction of it.

Regardless of the severity of the injury, it is vital to have a case manager involved as soon as possible. The case manager will be able to see 'the big picture' and will co-ordinate all aspects of the survivor's care. It will be the case manager who helps the survivor and the family 'navigate the system.' This is necessary because often the survivor and family will become involved not only with the health care system but also with insurance companies, lawyers, schools and training centres, and so on. The case manager will help the survivor and family work through a complex, fragmented, and often confusing array of programs. In a recent study of the service needs of brain injury survivors and their families, clients were asked, 'In looking back to the time of injury, what would have helped you deal with the situation?' The single most common answer was this: 'To have someone there, from the beginning, who would have explained things to us, helped us find the services needed, and explained the options to us.'

Survivors very often have memory loss, and suffer from confusion and from other symptoms that prevent them from absorbing the information provided about care options, and from making informed decisions. In some situations a family member will be able to provide 'case management' functions. However, families very often don't appreciate the seriousness of what has happened, and don't understand the health care system, and are very busy in their own lives while trying to do as much as possible for the injured family member. This is why a case manager is needed from the beginning to assist in co-ordinating care. The nearest office of any Brain Injury Association or Society can usually recommend a case manager (see Appendix A for information on brain injury associations).

After an Accident

Following are several scenarios of what happens after an accident resulting in brain injury. Some brain-injured survivors will experience only one or two of these scenarios; many others will experience several at various stages of recovery.

SCENARIOS:

1. Visit family doctor the same or next day.
2. Discharged home from the Emergency Department after a few hours or, at the most, twenty-four hours' observation.

3. Discharged home from hospital after several days or weeks.
4. Discharged from acute care to acute rehabilitation (the rehabilitation unit may be attached to the same hospital, or may be a free-standing rehabilitation centre).
5. Discharged to a slower-paced rehabilitation unit.
6. Discharged to a transitional living program.
7. Discharged to an extended care unit.

Very broadly speaking, these are the seven scenarios following injury. Now we will look at each of these seven scenarios a little more closely.

Scenario 1 Being involved in a relatively minor accident and seeing the family doctor the same day or next day can lead to some very frustrating problems if symptoms persist and there are indications of a mild traumatic brain injury. One of the top three complaints from survivors and their families is the lack of knowledge family doctors have about mild traumatic brain injury.

Scenario 2 The injured person is often discharged from the emergency department after only a few hours, without any information being given to the injured person or to the family. This can result in a great deal of confusion and anger, and have dangerous consequences.

Scenario 3 Discharge to home after a few days or weeks in hospital is far too often a terrible experience, and in some cases leaves scars that last a very, very long time. Indeed, I have seen cases where these scars lasted a lifetime. Little if any information is given to families, who assume that the injured family member must be 'okay,' since the decision was made to discharge him or her from the hospital.

Scenario 4 After a number of weeks or months, the individual is transferred to an active rehabilitation program. In the program, information and education specific to brain injury is likely to be provided to the family. Even so, far too often there are gaps in that information.

Scenario 5 The decision to discharge the survivor to a slower-paced rehabilitation centre is not always explained clearly to the survivor or the family. Why is the survivor not being discharged to a facility where he or she can be involved in a more active program?

Scenario 6 The reasons for discharge to a transitional living program are all too often unclear to families and survivors. Information is poorly explained to them, and alternatives are not discussed.

Scenario 7 Discharge to an extended care unit is often a heart-wrenching move for the family of a person with brain injury. An extended care facility is an inappropriate placement, especially if a young person is being placed with elderly people. While there may be few alternatives to extended care, far too often the ones that *are* available are not explored or fully explained.

The Case Manager

In all of the scenarios described above, a case manager is invaluable in co-ordinating the care of the survivor.

Initial phase In the initial stages after the injury, the case manager functions as another pair of ears for the family. He or she attends all meetings, supplements the information provided at these meetings, and asks the appropriate questions of those involved with the individual's care and rehabilitation.

At all times the case manager works closely with the family and the facility; the focus is on *representing and supporting the injured person*. The case manager helps the family make informed decisions, brings the family to look at other facilities, discusses their role in rehabilitation, and ensures that in the long run, the injured person is provided with the best opportunities available to become as independent as possible within the constraints of any ongoing disabilities. Many facilities have internal case managers, and while they do work with families, their obligation is to their employer, whether or not that employer is the provider of the service. An *independent* case manager is not affiliated in any way with anyone, and is there strictly to *work with the injured individual and family.*

The community Ideally, the same case manager should be involved from acute care right through to the person's return to the community, and then on a lifetime follow-up basis. Once the survivor is out of acute care and rehabilitation and into the community, the case manager ensures that the services being provided are in the best interests of the injured person and the family, and intervenes in the event of any personality conflicts, and sees that changes are made as needed in either personnel, or providers, or the overall program.

The case manager should be an authority on all the benefits that may be available to the injured person, and should advocate for services needed. For example, most brain injury survivors suffer from depression at some time during their recovery, yet some mental health providers feel that a head-injured person is inappropriate for their services. A case manager who notices signs of depression should refer the survivor to professionals who are specifically trained in diagnosing and treating depression (these include physicians, psychiatrists, and psychologists). Symptoms of depression that a case manager or family member might notice include a persistent sad or hopeless mood, eating irregularities, sleep disturbances, loss of energy, and slowing of speech or movement. These symptoms are often also present as symptoms of the brain injury, so if depression is suspected, it is important for the case manager to arrange for the survivor to see a mental health specialist. The specialist can determine whether the survivor's symptoms are a result of the injury, or are symptoms of 'down' or 'blue' days that we all experience, or are symptoms of *clinical depression,* which is a mental health condition that responds to proper treatment.

After fifteen years' experience as an independent case manager and over thirty years working with individuals who suffered catastrophic-type injuries, I am convinced that independent case managers, who can be arranged through nonprofit organizations such as state and provincial brain injury associations, provide a valuable service. None of us expect to be involved in an automobile crash resulting in serious injuries, and none of us expect to sustain any kind of injury, particularly a brain injury; and none of us are aware of how even a minor impact can cause brain damage and a lifetime of deficits. None of us know what questions to ask or how to deal with the information that doctors give us. We expect the doctor to have all the answers and that they will be correct.

There is research showing that families do not take in a great deal of information immediately after an injury, even when the information is made available to them. At workshops I have conducted involving families and survivors, the most typical comment I hear is that if they had had more information and education at the beginning, they would have done better, and they would have had fewer frustrations, and they would not have felt so alone in their struggles. This applies to the person who is in a coma for a month, as well as to the person who was unconscious for minutes. If case managers were made available through a provincial or state brain injury association *immediately for all families and survivors*, a great many ongoing problems would be prevented. The case manager would become involved initially at the hospital, being there to obtain information for the family, and to reinforce the information given to them, and would continue along these lines throughout the process. This could only be possible at hospitals that were willing to make immediate contact with the association for each new patient admitted with a brain injury. The original case manager would take the survivor through the various stages and back to the community from the hospital. If the individual's community was in another part of the province or state, a case manager from that community would take over, after becoming thoroughly familiar with the case.

The long-term role The case manager's hours of involvement will always be greater in the early stages. In the longer term, he or she may do much more than monitor the support services in place for the injured person. In some situations the only person involved from a support standpoint, other than the family, will be the case manager. The case manager may well become involved if the individual gets tied up with the court system for some reason or other. Inquiries may come from survivors when a cheque expected in the mail or into a bank account does not arrive. There could well be times when purchases were made that the individual could not afford, and negotiations will have to be made with the store or some other salesperson. The case manager may not be able to solve all of these difficulties, but he or she should be able to locate the sources of these problems.

Children   When the brain-injured person is a child or adolescent, the need for a case manager is at least as great, if not greater. For children and adolescents, the maze of questions, needs, and services can be even more confusing. Much of the extra confusion will relate to educational needs. The case manager will often help line up education consultants, and locate modified school programs, to ensure that the family and the child are fully supported and have the best possible opportunity in the school system. Still later, vocational training may need to be arranged.

7. Long-term Adjustment Following Significant Brain Injury

Mary Pepping, PhD

Once the initial flurry of emergency room and critical care has subsided, people with significant brain injury* usually enter a period of acute hospitalization. Then they are either discharged home with some professional assistance, or are transferred for some days or weeks to an in-patient rehabilitation unit.

Generally, after consistent improvements in mobility and communication are demonstrated, brain-injured survivors return home, where they receive some amount of follow-up and out-patient rehabilitation. Over time, as the involvement of professional staff begins to taper off, survivors and their families find themselves faced with the burden and challenge of coping with lifelong residual abilities and deficits.

In this chapter we will provide a summary of what has been learned over the past two decades about adjustment following significant brain injury. Specific suggestions for coping with the various issues that arise will also be discussed.

---

*In this context, *significant brain injury* refers to those injuries that result in twenty-four hours or greater loss of consciousness, and/or to the effects of a major stroke or other serious illness with known effects upon the brain (e.g., a brain tumour).

Typical Post-injury Changes in Function That People Must Face

In a person who has suffered a significant brain injury, likely to be encountered are some persistent changes in *thinking* (examples: reduced memory, and reduced speed of thinking), *personality* (heightened irritability, reduced capacity for empathy), *communication* (a tendency to stray from the topic at hand, word-finding difficulties), and *physical capacities* (changes in co-ordination, strength, and speed of movement). Such long-term general difficulties tend to be present whether the injured person has other residual problems or not.

Clearly, problems such as these can have an enormous impact on the capacity to work, and to love, successfully. They can also greatly affect the pleasure a person takes in life. It is important to note that there is plenty of room for individual uniqueness. No two people have *exactly* the same kinds of problems and abilities, either pre-injury or post-injury.

Consider, for example, two people who have moderate memory difficulties. One of them may be able to learn new information if it is presented in brief written form and is well-organized, and if given an opportunity to practise or rehearse it. The other person may not be able to recall information in word form, but if shown a picture or design may be able to retain that kind of information. So visual cues may work very well as reminders for this second person, for whom a picture truly is worth a thousand words.

Knowing and understanding the specific nature of someone's abilities and difficulties is critical to good long-term planning and adjustment. This is especially true for people with significant brain injury. People with brain injury not only need to relearn how to walk and talk during their early stages of recovery, but must also become reacquainted with many aspects of their new, or modified, self.

Some Important Questions

In order to predict, or appreciate, the long-term pattern of abilities and deficits that a specific individual is likely to manifest in the months and years following a brain injury, it helps to consider the following three questions.

1. What were the survivor's pre-injury assets and liabilities?

Any abilities and deficits that predate an injury will be a significant factor in long-term adjustment. In general, the greater the survivor's individual talents, and the fewer serious problems that person had prior to injury, the better he or she is likely to cope with a serious brain injury.

The following are some practical questions a friend, or family member, or person with brain injury, might ask in this regard:

- Was the person a good worker?
- Did the person get along well with other people?
- How did the person do in school?
- How well educated was the person?
- What had the person accomplished in life at the time of the accident?
- What was the person's pre-injury character?
- Could you count on the person to be responsible, to be caring?
- Did the person tend to have 'a short fuse,' or was he or she the kind of person who took a long time to get angry about something?

Everything you know about the person's pre-injury self will be important for understanding and helping the 'new' person who is emerging following the trauma. From a practical standpoint, it is a good idea to draw up a list of abilities and deficits that were always true of the person, and use that as a starting point for evaluating the post-injury situation.

2. How severe was the brain injury, and what are the specific changes in function the survivor must manage?

These changes tend to be categorized within the following areas:

- Thinking abilities and deficits.
- Personality and interpersonal issues.
- Communication disturbances, whether subtle or obvious.

- Physical capacities and limitations, both gross and fine.
- Vocational assets and liabilities.

In each of these areas of function, thorough re-evaluations conducted one year to eighteen months after injury will provide excellent information on likely long-term residual weaknesses and strengths.

If new problems arise, or if a person is a number of years post-injury and is not coping well, a review of progress made and needs still to be met is a good idea. Establishing an ongoing relationship with a managing physician, a nurse practitioner, a psychologist, or a rehabilitation case manager will maximize the survivor's chances of getting timely and appropriate assistance.

3. What are the survivor's emotional reactions to the injury?

And how well is the survivor able to cope with the resulting changes? Both these factors are of paramount importance in long-term adjustment. So are the *family's* emotional reactions and ability to deal with the stress of the situation.

Sometimes heightened emotional reactions and difficulties in adjusting become increasingly obvious during rehabilitation activities, especially those conducted on an out-patient or at-home basis. A survivor can become quite upset when first confronting his or her deficits. This is sometimes confusing to families, because after the early agitation associated with coming out of coma has subsided, many people with brain injury go through a period of rapid improvement, and do so quite calmly and with a positive outlook. Often during the early stages of recovery, the survivor is not fully aware of any deficits and may actually be less upset than the family about the injury and the difficulties arriving from it. At that point, survivors don't fully appreciate what is wrong, and what the implications may be for his or her work and personal life.

Later in recovery, survivors may become quite depressed, or anxious, or demoralized. Over time survivors must learn to strike a balance: they must be aware of any changes in ability and willing to accept them, without feeling too overwhelmed by them, and without minimizing them too much. An inability or refusal to find this balance can become a major stumbling block to progress. At other times, it is the family that may not be able to accept what is now different, or that may not be able to cope with the resulting differences in ability, character, job status, and/or productivity. These problems in coping are all completely normal, and those involved should obtain the services of the rehabilitation team members and/or a case manager who is familiar with brain injury and its effects. The supports or interventions that would be most helpful at that time can then be determined.

For example, a depressed mood can make a big difference in productivity; if this is the situation, a psychiatrist can be consulted, who might prescribe medications. Or if someone has become very withdrawn and physically deconditioned as well, a brief but well-organized set of activities, designed and supervised by a physical therapist and occupational therapist, may serve as a 'booster shot,' even when formal rehabilitation is some months or years in the past.

There are several additional areas we need to explore in long-term adjustment.

The Importance of Long-term Support for Survivors and Their Families

People with brain injury often need more support, and more structured follow-up over the years, than do people with other kinds of severe injuries. For example, people who have had spinal cord injuries, or severe burns, may need periodic physical check-ups over the years, to make sure that all their internal and external organs are working properly. However, they may not need much added help when changing jobs or coping with a family crisis.

The ability to think clearly and to manage emotional reactions appropriately makes a huge difference in long-term adjustment. A person or family that is facing life after significant brain injury will have to confront long-term permanent changes in these abilities.

There are often major changes in the roles and responsibilities individuals hold within the family. A parent who sustains a brain injury may be unable to work for a period for time; the other parent, and even adolescent children within the family, may have to take on full- or part-time work. Children may also have to take on additional household responsibilities. If a brother or sister is hurt, both parents may be very involved with the injured child for an extensive period of time, and this may affect how much time and attention the other children receive.

In the process of coping with these types of changes, family members may have to expand or shrink their earlier roles in ways that may lead to some permanent changes in family dynamics. Families may find that tasks such as paying bills, planning and organizing children's activities, and initiating social contact with friends have been reassigned within the family. Sometimes families discuss these changes directly, and sometimes they don't. The point is that changes of this magnitude are likely to have a strong impact on everyone.

During these difficult times, family members often find it helpful to seek out some therapy for themselves as individuals. Rehabilitation team members, the survivor's case manager, and the survivor's doctors can help them find family counselling or therapy. Family members may also benefit from support groups (discussed in chapter 15).

What Factors Predict Successful Long-term Adjustment?

Research has pinpointed several factors that predict healthy adjustment. These are all discussed below.

THE OVERALL SEVERITY OF THE BRAIN INJURY

When people have had very severe brain injuries, and have suffered profound changes in their ability to speak, or think, or behave appropriately, or move around freely, their ability to work and even to have fun with friends is often severely restricted. For these individuals a 'good outcome' may simply be that they can make eye contact with someone who loves them, or have improved some aspect of their basic communication, or perhaps (with the help of medication)

are less prone to serious seizures or to uncontrolled behavioural outbursts.

However, there is a large group of survivors who recover well
enough to be employable and live rich lives. One-third of people
who have been unconscious for twenty-four hours or longer after a
traumatic brain injury will resume some form of productive, paid
employment, on their own, after discharge from hospital. The
job may not be as complex, demanding or well paid as the one
held prior to the brain injury, but these people do return to the work
force and are able to cope with the day-to-day demands of being
productive.

Some survivors require intensive out-patient rehabilitation programs after discharge, before they are able to resume work and a
productive life. About half of survivors of severe brain injury return
to full-time work following rehabilitation.

ADDITIONAL FACTORS CRITICAL TO ADJUSTMENT

Although the overall severity of a person's injury certainly makes
a difference to his or her ability to work and relate to others, there
are additional considerations. The people who are most *capable* of
doing some kind of work after injury, are not necessarily those
with the highest intelligence. The ones who are successful at work,
and at home with family and friends, tend to exhibit the following
characteristics:

- They are aware of their personal abilities and deficits following
  the injury.
- They are able to accept that there has been some change in ability
  that will likely result in some change in job status.
- They are willing to use compensatory techniques (such as a memory book, a Daytimer schedule, or a double-checking system) to
  maintain or improve daily performance.
- They can get along reasonably well with other people.
- They are able to maintain a sense of hope – to believe that life can
  improve.

These factors are the best predictors of who will have a positive, productive life following a brain injury.

Can We Foster Development of These Critical Factors?

Many people who have been brain injured are capable of developing greater awareness and acceptance of their condition; they are also capable of improving their ability to compensate for their deficits and to get along well with other people. In this process, a sense of hope often develops, as the person notices his or her own improvement.

Even people who are two years post-injury – which is part the time when all spontaneous recovery is likely to occur – can profit from treatment in the critical areas noted above. If you have had a brain injury, and are struggling with these issues, even after the usual rehabilitation efforts you may well be a candidate for further treatment.

Who or What Can Help?

If a survivor of brain injury is capable of some kind of productive work, but faces problems that are obstacles to employment, a more intensive, milieu-based kind of treatment, with a strong return-to-work focus, may be indicated. Experienced rehabilitation teams that are familiar with the long-term challenges that face brain-injured people can be valuable allies in improving long-term adjustment at home, at work, and in the community. (Provided in chapter 4 was a description of the roles that different team members play.)

These rehabilitation teams may operate within out-patient departments and programs connected to hospitals, or they may be community-based programs, or they may be free-standing programs that deliver treatment 'in the field' – that is, within the home, or at the job site. The setting is not as important as the experience, philosophy, and 'team spirit' of the clinical staff.

When shopping for such programs, talk to the managers or clinical directors, and to some of their team members. Also, speak to former 'graduates' of the treatment and ask them about the progress they made while in the program. What kinds of people, of what ages and backgrounds and occupations, tend to do well in the program? Does it seem like a good fit with what you need?

Such teams can also be invaluable in letting you know what is (or is not) realistic and appropriate at a particular point in time post-injury. They can help make realistic plans that allow for periodic revision according to accomplishments, needs, and circumstances.

Even with excellent staff and programs, and strong commitment and hard work on the part of the survivor and his or her family, not every brain-injured person is capable of resuming full-time employment. But part-time employment, or the development of volunteer work placements, or other improvements in function and coping, are all within the proper scope of treatment.

What Do Employers Think Is Important for Long-term Success?

In looking at the larger question of return to productivity, and to work if possible, it is very instructive to interview employers, and others who have supervised people with or without brain injuries. Employers are quite consistent in their descriptions of what is required to be a good employee. These descriptions typically include the following traits:

- Gets to work on time, and every day.
- Has good basic personal hygiene – is clean and neat.
- Knows how to do the task, is accurate and timely.
- Asks questions when necessary, but not constantly.
- Works at a steady pace – doesn't 'goof off' or waste time, and doesn't distract other employees from their work.
- Can be counted on to do what is asked.
- Gets along well with other employees, and with the boss.

Employers are also quick to point out that these are qualities they would want to see in *any* employee, brain-injured or not. In many instances these supervisors were willing to consider hiring someone who might need modifications to the workplace, who would need a job coach for a while, and who might take longer to learn a new task (or need to keep a memory book handy), provided that person could meet the seven qualifications listed above in a reasonable period of time.

There are certainly many exceptions to this positive attitude on the part of employers. In general, studies of long-term employment after brain injury reveal that for survivors who are capable of paid work, problems in finding or maintaining suitable employment have three basic causes:

1. Residual behavioural problems that adversely affect interpersonal skills.
2. Difficulty accepting a lower level of job status or income if the severity of the brain injury makes it impossible for the person to return to the previous level of employment.
3. Once employed, trouble adapting to subsequent major changes in job duties or requirements, without some added help.

Among people who are considered capable of working after brain injury, it isn't a specific kind of memory problem, or language deficit, or problem-solving impairment per se, that ultimately determines success. Rather, it is the survivor's emotional and interpersonal abilities and attitudes that seem to make the critical difference in successful long-term adjustment.

The Role of Financial Disincentives

Finally, if there are powerful financial incentives to remain 100 per cent disabled or impaired, brain-injured people may find it almost impossible to risk competitive employment. This is especially true if their families do not want them to work, for fear of losing disability income, or for fear of jeopardizing the size of any financial settlement in a legal case. As a result, these individuals may go on to lead more restricted lives than is necessary.

The long-term negative impact of such restrictions can greatly exacerbate the losses in self-esteem and self-worth that often accompany significant brain injury.

Love, Relationships, Family, and Friends

One of the most critical factors in successful long-term adjustment is the nature of family relationships and support. Families of people who have sustained significant brain injury face an especially painful and persistent long-term challenge. The survivor may have changed dramatically since the injury, and family and friends may have a difficult time adjusting to this changed person.

Changes in Personality and Behaviour Important changes in personality and behaviour following damage to the brain can create 'a different person.' Living with this 'new person' is often a very daunting task for family and friends. On top of this, the sometimes dimly felt, sometimes acutely felt, change in *sense of self* brings many brain-injured people to the brink of personal despair.

Families and friends sometimes report that the person who has had the brain injury is now nicer than he or she had been prior to the injury. This is the exception rather than the rule. That being said, changes in the brain's frontal lobe functions sometimes lead a person to be more expressive of affection, or more 'easy going,' than before the injury. This might be a welcome change for family and friends, especially if the person was very quiet, or shy, or overly anxious and worried, prior to the injury.

Generally, however, the changes in personality that occur following damage to the frontal, temporal, or parietal lobes lead to problems. These problems include increased irritability, misperception of other people's intentions and comments, a tendency to be self-centred, a reduction in the ability to empathize with others, a decline in the ability to understand what is happening and what is needed in a particular social situation, inappropriate comments or behaviour (for example, asking people rude questions), an inability to 'read' other people's emotions, and uncontrolled laughing or crying.

These factors can all lead to uncomfortable, frustrating, and dissatisfying interactions, which can become even more wearing and wearying over time. One of the toughest realities that brain-injured people and their families must face is the degree of social withdrawal, social abandonment, and social isolation that occurs following significant brain injury.

Reactions of Friends and Family in Long-term Adjustment Old friends may stop coming by, because they do not feel comfortable with the mental, emotional, and/or physical changes they can now see in their brain-injured friend. Or these old friends may be busy with their own lives. Also, if the person with brain injury is no longer at work or school, then the opportunity for contact that was present before, disappears.

The family may also find itself increasingly isolated, with less time and energy for outside pursuits, and less comfort inviting friends over for dinner or coffee. Common as well is some degree of personal depression, sadness, and fatigue, which saps family members' own levels of interest and energy.

Very loyal or compassionate friends, especially long-term ones, sometimes remain, but most other pre-injury social contacts tend to diminish or change over time. In this kind of circumstance a number of pro-active steps can be taken, both for the family and for the person with brain injury.

What Can Be Done to Reclaim a Meaningful Life?

The following suggestions are offered to the survivor to assist in reclaiming a meaningful life:

- Become aware of your residual strengths and weaknesses; compensate for the problems, and appreciate what you have to offer people vis-à-vis your strengths.
- Get involved in support groups, for example, through your national or local Brain Injury Association, and make some new friends there, among people who may have a better understanding of the challenges you are facing.
- Get involved in work or volunteer activities, which not only bring you into contact with other people, but give you some common topics of interest and day-to-day experience to discuss.

- If you belong to a church community, find out if there are special events or activities for persons with disabilities.
- Take a class at your local community college. When registering, ask the Student Services department whether there are special instructors or tutors or groups on campus, that help people with disabilities enjoy the classroom and campus environment.
- Follow a good exercise program, within your abilities. This will help you manage stress and increase your energy.
- Establish regular sleep and eating habits.
- Follow a regular daily schedule that includes plans for carrying out household and community tasks and activities.
- Learn to use public transportation, if driving is not an option.

The above is not an exhaustive list, but it is a good beginning for the process of reclaiming one's sense of place, and meaning.

After any crisis or tragedy, people must often face 'starting over.' After a brain injury, it can be especially difficult to independently generate ideas for problem solving, and follow through effectively, while maintaining one's mood and equanimity. With help, it is certainly possible. Family members' contributions in this regard, and rehabilitation professionals' initial and periodic input, will be important factors in long-term success.

Is There a Silver Lining to This Cloud?

The ability to work and be productive, and the ability to love and get along well with others, and the ability to relax and have fun, are all integral to a sense of meaning and happiness. For successful, long-term adjustment after someone in the family has sustained a significant brain injury, personal, family, and professional efforts must be directed toward achieving these goals.

The obstacles to achieving these three broad goals (to *work*, to *love*, to *have fun*) will of course vary with the age and capacities of the survivor. Certainly, the needs of young children will differ from those of mature adults. It is probably safe to say, however, that in all circumstances it will be terribly overwhelming to face such changes, such challenges, and such upheaval.

Good long-term adjustment is most possible if we view the process of rehabilitation and recovery as ongoing and life-long. Achieving self-improvement, learning how to cope, practising new ways of being the person we have become, and exploring new forms of leisure are necessary for all of us, but especially for those who are recovering from brain injury.

Such flexibility does not come easily for anyone. For those who are learning to live with brain injury, periodic professional contact, advice, and support will always be important. Rehabilitation professionals in your area can help you locate the specific kinds of help you need, at the times you need it.

For some people, the experience of coping with brain injury, whether as a survivor or a family member or friend, will have some positive aspects in the long term. These can include the following:

- A clearer or deeper realization of how precious life can be.
- A very great appreciation of the importance of family and friends.
- A reordering of priorities in life, so that one takes more time to be with friends and family rather than working a sixty-hour week.
- Pursuit of hobbies and interests that have been 'put off' for too long.
- A greater sense of compassion for other people in the world, and the community.

Finally, some American studies reveal that people with brain injury are much more likely to volunteer their time to various charitable or educational causes. This, even among those who are working regularly.

8. 'Rime' of the Survivor

David Blanche, BRe

What can a survivor of brain injury tell someone about this trauma? The best way to describe what it is like to have a brain injury is to introduce my constant companion since 1973 – an albatross.

'The Rime of the Ancient Mariner' by Samuel Taylor Coleridge is an epic poem about a ship sailing between Africa and South America that is caught in the doldrums. The wicked old captain, the 'ancient mariner,' and his disgruntled crew are as restless in spirit as their ship is calm.

After several days a bird with a huge wingspan, an albatross, appears and circles the ship. The crew know the albatross bears good luck and feel blessed by its presence. The angry captain, however, resenting the crew's jubilant mood, goes below deck, returns with a crossbow, and shoots the bird. The crew are upset, and seek a punishment that fits the mariner's crime. So they shackle the albatross to his neck. The ancient mariner returns to the world with the corpse hanging from his neck, marked for life like a cast-out leper.

In many ways, I feel like that ancient mariner: there is an albatross around my neck too. When I began recovering from my accident, it would hang in front of my legs, tripping me up when I tried to move forward. I would fall, both metaphorically and literally. I often stumbled and hurt myself. To this day, I still bear some emotional and physical scars. The early stages of my recovery were the most difficult: sometimes, the pain was overwhelming. I had not asked for this punishment, nor did I deserve it. I could not understand. I might have broken down completely – but I had forgotten how to cry. I did not know what to do or where to go. Could this be life?

My name is David Blanche and I am a survivor of brain injury. In 1973, when I was an eighteen-year-old high school student, a car accident left me unconscious for thirty-two days and paralysed my right side.

As a result of this accident, my old self died and was replaced by a new self. I underwent what I refer to as a 'change of self.' This concept is difficult to seize, even for the person who undergoes the change. Everything I know how to do today I have learned at least twice. I had grown to a nearly mature eighteen-year-old, died as a result of a brain injury, and was reborn. I had to learn again all of those things I already knew, as well as grow to be a man.

This rebirth was followed by *confusion* – I did not know who I was. When I left the acute care hospital after three months, I was excited about re-entering my old life. But there was one thing I could not see: *I had changed.* I was not the same person I had been before the accident. I did not walk the same, talk the same, or think the same. I was different. It was hard for me to recognize this at the time. My parents could see it but I could not and no one told me I was different. I felt like this new kid in the crowd, only this new kid was not wanted.

About this time my thought processes and memory were starting to work on their own and a realization came to me. My physical recovery from the accident was slowing down. I was not progressing as fast as I had been only a month before. Maybe I would not be completely cured in a few months. During this time failure seemed to follow failure. I lost my girlfriend and my other friends. I was failing at school. Before the accident I had been an athlete. Now I lost my shape and my self-image. I felt like I was lost in space, walking around in a world where nobody knew or understood who I was. I needed someone to help me, but there was no one. I remember one day walking as far as I could and not talking to anyone along the way and no one talking to me.

I touched bottom during those days. It was like being stuck down a deep well. It was so deep that if I looked up, all I could see through the darkness was a speck of light. I was alone and had doubts about reaching that light.

By then I knew there was something wrong with me, but I did not know what it was. I had no insight or understanding of my brain injury and did not know what to do. The health care professionals did not seem to know much about this aspect of brain injury. When I re-entered my old life I found I did not fit in. Failure and rejection followed me around during my first years as a survivor. I missed people – friends talking, laughing, smiling. I felt that no one loved me. *Loneliness* was constant. I needed others but my desperation only caused further rejection. I tried to think about what to do. Answers came from everybody: do this, try that, come here, go there, stop, don't do that. I was very confused.

I did not know who I was, so I went in search of my elusive self. I tried to go back to school. That year at college, I took five courses, dropped three and barely passed two. Being persistent, I tried college for three more semesters with similar results before I decided that college was not for me.

I thought I should get a job. I spent a lot of time looking for a position, with limited success. Finally I found work in the warehouse of the Liquor Control Board (now the Liquor Distribution Branch), unloading large containers. It was a backbreaking, mindless job, but I thought I could do it. After about a week, the supervisor called me into his office. I thought he was going to be angry with me for taking too long in the washroom, but instead he told me, 'We don't have any place for a cripple here.'

For a moment, I did not know whom he was referring to. I did not see myself as a cripple. Then I realized he was talking about me. I left feeling numb, curiously detached from the rest of the world.

Again I did not know where to go or what to do. I did not know what was happening to me. One of the things the Liquor Control Board supervisor had mentioned was to see my family doctor. But I was not ill, so why bother him? I stood outside that warehouse for a long time. I thought, maybe the doctor could do something.

Still feeling numb, I went to the doctor's office where I felt alone in a room full of people. The doctor saw me and I told him what had happened. He listened. He said he thought his friend could help. I could not think of anything else to do so I went to see his friend.

This man – a psychiatrist, I suppose – was friendly. He spoke with a German accent and asked me if I liked men or women, if I masturbated, if I liked my mother. I could not see how these questions related to my problem. I did not have a job and did not know where to look for one. What did my mother have to do with my problems?

We got past that line of questioning and began to talk. He said that I was never going to be a labourer. I would have to do something with my head. I felt lost and agreed with this man who seemed to hold a ray of hope. We agreed I should start at a community college and develop sufficient skills and knowledge to enter university. My new doctor also got me in touch with a government organization called 'Aid to the Handicapped,' which eventually paid for two years of community college and three years of university. After many interviews and testing sessions, the consensus was that I should study 'Recreation Education.'

Over the next five years I pursued this goal and graduated in 1981 with a bachelor's degree in Recreation Education. Earning this degree taught me a great deal and helped fill the void created by my 'change of self' experience. Although I still did not feel that I fit into the real world, I felt successful from having reached a goal.

I held many jobs during this period, but none for more than a few months. I worked in the fields of geriatrics and mental disabilities and felt a real need to help. Nevertheless, after a few years, I still felt that something was missing. At this stage, I tried to understand what I needed to do to be fulfilled. Feeling a great need to work more closely with people and help with human issues, I decided that either social work or counselling psychology was where I needed to be. I returned to university to take courses which were prerequisites for both fields. By the end of a year I decided that social work was the path I ought to take.

In 1986, I entered the social work program full of excitement and expectations. During the first few months of class, I had a work placement where I worked with brain injured adults. I had a feeling that I knew what they were talking about because I shared some of the same experiences. I realized that the experiences of my own injury could help others in their recovery. The potential for fulfilment excited me. I thought I had found my place.

I finished the course work but had trouble with my work placement. I am not sure what happened but I failed that part of my social work course. I fought to get another placement but failed that one too. I felt devastated. The goal that I had set was slipping away and I felt helpless again.

During this program, I did make an important discovery. I had been thinking that, as a consequence of my car accident, I had undergone an experience that no one else had gone through or could relate to. Meeting other brain injured people made me feel part of a group; I was no longer alone. I also discovered professionals who worked with brain-injured people and better understood what I had gone through. I discovered support groups and advocacy and information organizations for brain injured people.

As I met other brain injury survivors, I learned about the range of causes and the severity of their traumas. I found out that some were wrestling with insurance and compensation claims, something I had never had to do.

A few uncomfortable months after failing to pass the social work program, I decided to use the knowledge and skills that I had learned to help other brain-injured people. Since then I have tried to help people who suffer from brain injuries. I had valuable assets: I had professional training in social work and counselling, as well as having survived brain injury myself. The lack of a social work degree, however, and the cognitive deficits that I still have, have so far prevented me from living up to my personal expectations.

I have learned that I must adjust my personal goals to reality. Although I have conditioned my body to a high level of fitness, I still have cognitive deficits that are as much a part of me as the colour of my eyes.

Still, my fate has been better than the ancient mariner's in Coleridge's poem. I no longer feel like I used to, in all senses of the word. I have learned to push my albatross from in front of my legs to a place near the centre of my back. But I still feel the weight of that bird. Sometimes, the albatross shifts, falls in front of my legs and trips me.

A problem with this weight is that no one can see it. Often, when I explain it to someone, I get a blank look in return. After all, I do not appear any different. And when you look normal, you are expected to act normal. For me, however, fulfilling these expectations can be a struggle. I want to continue progressing, however. My albatross is still there, an inescapable companion. But after all these years, I have learned to know and accept it. I shall continue following the course I embarked upon when I was reborn after the car accident.

9. Psychosocial Effects of Brain Injury

J. David Seaton

Philosopher William James once wrote that 'no more fiendish punishment could be devised than that one should be turned loose in society and remain absolutely unnoticed by all its members.' It is doubtful that he was referring to someone with a brain injury when he made this statement in the 1890s; even so, it well describes the struggle many brain-injured individuals experience in trying to regain a meaningful life. Until recent years it was usually the individual's physical limitations that were seen as the main obstacle preventing reintegration into the community. It is now recognized that psychosocial deficits present the greatest challenges for brain injury survivors.

A person with a brain injury is often described as 'not being the same' after the injury. This is mainly in reference to personality changes (that is, the way the person is expected to act relative to pre-injury behaviour). Generally, these changes are psychosocial in nature, and relate to the ability to develop and maintain meaningful relationships. Psychosocial deficits often result in the person having problems maintaining previous relationships and developing new relationships. It is not uncommon for someone with psychosocial deficits to eventually be alienated from others. This often results in the person with a brain injury becoming progressively more socially isolated, despondent, and dependent on immediate family members.

Physical deficits, while important, do not stigmatize the survivor nearly as much as behaviours such as staring, inappropriate language or humour, repeating oneself, impulsivity, bad temper, and poor judgment. Often, because an individual with a brain injury looks 'normal,' it is hard for others to understand that his or her social deficits are a result of injury and not evidence of psychological abnormality. Society has long shied away from and discriminated against individuals who are socially or behaviourally different. This is mainly due to our fear of their unpredictability, whether the cause is mental illness, or homelessness, or brain injury. It is easy for society to sympathize with someone who is in a wheelchair because of an injury, such as actor Christopher Reeves. It is harder for most people to comprehend that someone is 'acting different' because of an injury, as does James Brady, who was President Reagan's press secretary.

Brain injury is often referred to as the 'silent epidemic.' This is not only because of the rapidly growing number of cases, but also because most people in society simply fail to understand the severity and consequences of the disability.

Life-long Living

Brain injury happens mainly to young adults; an estimated 70 per cent of survivors are between 15 and 28 years old. It is anticipated that most of these young adults will live a normal life span, which means they will survive another fifty years with a chronic disability. It was believed back in the 1970s and early 1980s that a person with a brain injury had a window of recovery limited to twelve to eighteen months, after which little or no progress could be expected. After that time, formal rehabilitation was stopped, and most individuals were discharged either to home, or to a nursing facility or psychiatric hospital for custodial care. The belief that there was a 'plateau' to recovery became a self-fulfilling prophecy, since few people made additional progress once relegated to one of these socially deprived environments. However, with the emergence of non-institutionalized brain-injury treatment programs in the mid-1980s, learning theory and developmental treatment models have begun to replace the time-limited, medical model in brain injury rehabilitation. The approach these treatment models promote is that individuals with disabilities do *not* plateau – rather, *environments* do. From this assumption, it follows that progress is based on learning. The earlier, custodial approach focused on maintenance; the goal in brain injury rehabilitation is to create supportive and stimulating environments that foster ongoing growth and normalized living. People continue to grow and change throughout their life when they learn new skills and are given the opportunity to flourish.

It is commonly believed that people are successful because they are motivated. Actually, people are motivated because they are successful. Only individuals who experience more successes than failures can feel good about themselves. Unfortunately, on a daily basis, most individuals with a brain injury experience many more failures than successes because of their social and cognitive deficits. Example: a salesman was naturally able to think quickly, retain information, and present a charming personality to customers; after suffering a brain injury, he became frustrated and depressed about his inability to perform at previous levels.

The most common cognitive deficits that contribute to an individual's inability to function at pre-injury levels relate to planning, and to organizing information in a logical sequence, and to retaining information. These cognitive deficits are attributed to deficits in insight, initiation, judgment, and problem solving. The survivor is limited in the ability to make realistic plans, consider options, and predict the likely consequences of actions. As a result, the person with these deficits often experiences a more chaotic lifestyle, repeated failures, and diminished confidence.

Strategies for addressing these cognitive deficits include the following: (1) establishing consistent routines and structures in daily activities, (2) teaching the survivor to use compensatory cognitive aids, such as calendars and written daily plans, (3) developing approaches for dealing with breaks in routine and less familiar situations, and (4) helping the survivor 'over-learn' skills within a variety of different settings. By establishing a structured routine for someone with a brain injury, we create a more predictable environment; this in turn decreases confusion, agitation, and dependence.

Role of the Environment and Support

Brain injury rehabilitation programs are designed to improve an individual's functioning, with the expectation that once various skills are achieved they will be maintained in different environments. Sometimes, however, these skills cannot be maintained or generalized outside of a supportive environment. In other words, it is not uncommon for someone to regress after being discharged from a program.

This phenomenon has been noted for decades with the mentally ill. A person with mental illness will be admitted to a psychiatric hospital and make tremendous gains within the structured, supportive treatment setting, only to regress after being discharged. This process has been called the 'revolving door' syndrome, because the person may spend years, or even a lifetime, going in and out of hospitals without ever attaining a stable lifestyle. It is not recommended that someone spend an entire life in a treatment program in order to function at a higher level; but at the same time, it is crucial that some of the therapeutic ingredients found in the treatment setting be established in the post-discharge setting. For example, within the treatment setting the person may have an active, predictable schedule, and receive regular feedback from staff and peers. There may be rewards based on achievements, and the environment may be adjusted to accommodate the survivor's deficits (this is where calendars come in, as well as daily schedule cards and regular staff reminders). Too often, the person is discharged to a setting that has few if any of these environmental supports. Understandably, the person usually regresses outside the treatment setting. To minimize regression or setback, it is critical that as many of these environmental supports as possible be transferred from the treatment setting to the home.

A supportive environment, although not a cure-all, must be maintained in order to minimize the disability. A good analogy here is a pair of glasses: they help a person see better, without actually improving that person's eyes. Also, simply trying harder to see better without glasses does nothing to improve one's vision. The disability does not go away because of the glasses, but it is compensated for. In the same way, a supportive environment does not change the individual; rather, it allows that individual to compensate for the disability and improve his or her functioning level.

For most individuals with brain injury, memory and cognitive deficits are a major source of frustration and limitation. To help them compensate for these deficits, we must provide structure. *Structure* involves creating a routine that is predictable, and establishing daily activities in a set schedule that allows survivors to remember what they previously did and what they are going to do later in the day. Often a person with a brain injury has an unpredictable routine, because there is no longer a built-in structure of work and other obligations. So the person may stay up late, get up at different times, leave valuables in different places, eat meals whenever hungry, and so on.

Such people are often scattered, have poor recall of events, lose items, and easily become frustrated or agitated. A structure gives people a starting point and offers predictability for the day. But providing structured routines is usually not sufficient to address cognitive deficits. The person must also learn to use a variety of compensatory memory aids, which may be difficult since the person never used them previously. It is easy for us to take our memory for granted, but it is nearly always effected by a brain injury. Also, it is difficult for us to know what we have forgotten until it is pointed out by others, and this can cause embarrassment, frustration, and anger. For these reasons it is best for someone with a brain injury to develop a structured routine in which memory aids are used consistently.

Disability is amplified when the environment fails to support the individual's needs. Since the environment has such a pervasive effect on a disabled person's functioning level, the individual is no longer the sole focus of intervention. The environmental questions that must be considered in tandem with individual factors include these: Is there enough structure? Is there enough consistency? Is there enough repetition? Is there enough reward? Is there enough support? Is it specific enough? Is it practical? Is it meaningful?

A person with a brain injury may retain many cognitive skills, but may also have difficulty applying them, except in very familiar or routine settings. A structured environment and cognitive aid (such as a computer, or organizer, or notebook, or calendar) reduce the demand on cognitive functioning. People with brain injury must make compensatory skills a regular part of their life if they wish to experience greater success and achieve more independence.

Self-esteem and Success

People who feel good about themselves usually have good lives. Unfortunately, the converse is also true. How we feel about ourselves significantly effects virtually every aspect of our functioning; it follows that self-esteem is the key to our success or failure. Self-esteem is created through feelings of personal competence and personal worth. It is associated with our most desirable attributes, such as empathy and altruism, and also with undesirable behaviours such as egocentrism and aggression.

Humans are social animals by nature, and for most people relationships are a key to feeling important and connected to the world. Relationships with family members are usually quite important; however, most people derive many of their social relationships from those with whom they work and play. After a brain injury, individuals are often much less socially integrated, and feel like outsiders in society because they cannot reintegrate into the many social roles they once played.

The need to feel important – to *matter* – is at the core of human emotions. Unfortunately, those who perceive that it is not possible to matter in a positive way, are likely to find other ways to feel they matter. Out of the need to feel important, people may develop more acting out behaviours, such as joining a gang, allowing themselves to be exploited by others, and developing attention-seeking behaviours (aggression, yelling, self-abuse, and so on).

A major challenge for caregivers after a brain injury is to find ways to reintegrate the survivor with a variety of positive social opportunities. The following everyday activities can help promote relationships for individuals with brain injury: performing volunteer work, joining sports or interest clubs, attending church, taking classes, using chat rooms on the Internet, and joining community organizations and civic groups. Being a part of society means contributing to it and participating in the available resources. Being a part of a larger group helps people to develop a sense of community, and to feel that they *do* matter and are part of society. This in turn, helps reduce feelings of isolation; it also fosters self-esteem.

Substance Abuse and Brain Injury

A person who feels rejected, unaccepted, or unloved is easily exploited by others. Such people very often gravitate to the use of alcohol or drugs in the hope of deadening their emotional pain. In a national survey on alcohol abuse and brain injury, one respondent with a brain injury answered that he drank because 'I can't do anything about the disability, but I can about the pain.' Because it is legal, affordable, accessible, and predictable in its results, alcohol is the leading form of substance abuse. In addition, what may have not been considered a drinking problem before the injury (perhaps a couple of beers after work, or wine with dinner), may now be a problem because even this minimal intake exacerbates the cognitive, physical, and behavioural deficits arising from the brain injury.

It is unlikely for someone with a brain injury who abuses alcohol or drugs to stop unless provided with some meaningful reason why, and with something to replace what was offered by alcohol or drugs. This is especially true when peer relations are associated with the abuse. Seldom does someone give up a behaviour unless it can be replaced with something equally or more rewarding. If they are to have a life free of alcohol and drugs, people with a brain injury absolutely must begin to establish an active daily schedule that fills in free time. They must set attainable goals, experience daily successes, and develop alternative friends, such as in a support group, church, or club.

Behaviour and Reinforcement

Most behaviours can be placed in these three categories: attention seeking, avoidance, and wanting something. If a behaviour achieves a goal, the person is more likely to use that behaviour again in similar situations. For example, everyone has witnessed a child crying for candy in a checkout line. The child usually keeps up this behaviour, increasing the volume of cries until the parent relents and gives the child the candy. The reason the child uses this behaviour is that it works. To develop an alternative behaviour, the parent must not reward the child for the original behaviour, but rather must reward the child for the behavior that *is* desired. This is not easy: in fact, at first the child may *increase* the old behaviour, since it worked well in the past. It will take time for the child to learn a new behaviour, but this will happen if real rewards are applied consistently. The following story highlights this phenomenon:

A weekend fisherman looked over the side of his boat and saw a snake with a frog in its mouth. Feeling sorry for the frog, he reached down and gently removed the frog from the snake's mouth and let the frog go free. But now he felt sorry for the hungry snake. Having no food, he took out his flask of bourbon and poured a couple of drops in the snake's mouth. The snake swam away happy, the frog was happy, and the fisherman was happy for doing such a good deed. After a few minutes had passed he heard a knock on the side of his boat. With stunned disbelief, the fisherman saw that the snake was back, this time with two frogs in his mouth.

The moral of the story is that you get what you reward. In trying to do the right thing, we often fall into the trap of rewarding the wrong behaviour and ignoring the right one.

In modifying behaviour, it is important to know what motivates the person. In other words, what are they willing to work for? It is important to discuss the reward plan with the person, and possibly even establish a written agreement or contract. The more black-and-white, or concrete, the plan is, the better. Behaviour modification should not be secretly executed on someone else. Rather, it is most effective when communicated openly and based on what the person is already motivated to achieve.

Learning and Progress

For change to occur, a person first has to accept that there needs to be change; second, that persons must be in a safe environment for change; and third, that person needs to develop new skills. People will not change any behaviour unless they perceive the problems associated with the behaviour and accept that the behaviour must be changed. People only 'experiment' with behaviour change when they feel safe enough to try new behaviours. Someone who is anxious or scared is unlikely to try something new, and likely to keep doing what he or she has always done. That is why it is so important to establish a consistent structure or routine, so that the person can predict both the environment and the outcome.

For change to occur, new skills must be learned. It is not simply a matter of being motivated, or of trying harder, or of the passage of time. 'Insanity' was once defined as doing the same thing over and over again and expecting a different result. Change requires developing new skills through practice. Thus, a person with a brain injury who wishes to improve his or her memory, will need to learn to use a notebook and calendar; to become stronger that person will need to exercise; to meet people that person will need to go where people are; to get a job that person will have to apply for work that is commensurate with existing skills and abilities.

A person who wishes to learn and make progress must be aware of the existing problem. Unfortunately, people with brain injury sometimes have limited insight into their behaviour. Increasing someone's awareness about their deficits is usually a double-edged sword, since most people feel more angry and depressed the more they understand about their loss. This cyclical process of anger and depression is actually a phase of recovery, and a normal grief reaction. Sometimes lack of insight is called 'denial.'

However, denial can also be seen as a 'psychological antibody' that protects the person from being bombarded by harsh realities. Most people cannot comprehend nor adequately deal with the enormous losses that brain injury involves. Thus, lack of insight may actually be a protective mechanism that enables the person to gradually absorb the realities of the situation at an acceptable rate. It is not necessarily helpful or advisable to force people to confront the realities of their loss. It is better to let people absorb these realities at their own pace.

It is not uncommon for someone with a brain injury to express feelings of helplessness and hopelessness. One of the most effective approaches to dealing with these emotions is to *do something*. This process of doing something, or *empowerment*, helps instil the feeling that there are again options and choices available in life. Empowerment fosters itself if the person is provided with encouragement and opportunity. It is a basic human instinct that gives people a sense of ownership of their own life. Empowerment expands as a person interacts and integrates in a variety of new experiences and begins to feel more connected to life. People who develop a strong sense of empowerment stop feeling like victims. They become accountable for their feelings and actions and find meaning and a will to live on. To become empowered, people need encouragement. Encouragement may be found in support groups with peers, in therapy, in self-help books, or through the support of friends and family.

The goal of brain injury rehabilitation is to help the individual live the highest quality of life possible. This can only be achieved through some degree of self-acceptance and a healthy self-esteem. For someone with a brain injury, a question that often arises is this: *How do I now fit into the world and what role do I play?* A new understanding of self is now needed. While honesty is usually the best policy, it is unwise to ever remove another person's hope and optimism that life can get better. Honesty is best conveyed in a supportive environment that encourages active participation and involvement. Within such an environment, people can continue to grow and change. Human beings are resilient. We make changes throughout our lives as we become motivated, develop the skills, and create the opportunities. These life changes may be losing weight, stopping smoking, going to school, running a marathon, learning a foreign language, or whatever our goal or dream may be at that time in our life.

When the student is ready, the teachers will appear. There are many mountains to overcome after a brain injury. The most important things that caregivers can offer in this process are support and encouragement. All people can and do continue to grow and change when they have the abilities to pursue life's opportunities. The only outcome that really matters in life, for anybody, is the ability to enjoy it.

10. Children and Adolescents with Brain Injury

Marilyn Unger, PhD

This chapter will briefly review some important information about children and adolescents with brain injury and the process of coping with their rehabilitation. Brain trauma is the leading cause of death in children and the most common cause of acquired disability. Approximately 1 in 500 children per year in the United States sustain a brain injury that results in a change in level of consciousness, or a physical abnormality of the brain, or both. Before the 1960s most children died after a serious traumatic brain injury (TBI). In Canada and the United States, as well as in other countries, advances in medical sciences have begun to save these children's lives. However, there has not been as much research on the effects of brain injury on children and youth as there has been on adults. The research that has been done shows more variability in both cognitive and behavioural difficulties than for adults.

Family members of brain-injured young people are likely to have been closely involved in the injury itself. Brain injuries of children and young people happen at home, in the local neighbourhood, while riding in the family car, or while crossing the street with family members. This may mean that other family members have been injured or killed. Because the child or adolescent is dependent on the family for support and training, the family is at the centre of the rehabilitation process. The significant disruption in the family's life caused by a child's brain injury may well result in some family members questioning their basic assumptions about life, happiness, success, and so on. This process of disruption often involves over-whelming emotions. If there are other children in the family, their lives are dramatically affected as well. In the early phases of the injury, some parents or other family members are in a state of shock. Many parents have symptoms associated with post-traumatic stress. They may be haunted by memories of the traumatic event and have sleep problems and increased anxiety levels.

It is more difficult for a family to specify how the brain injury has affected their child and to develop realistic expectations, because a child is not fully developed at the time of the injury. Ambiguity and uncertainty about the future hinder the parents' and family's process of adapting to the child's brain injury. It is important to remember that each family is different and that each family will cope with this difficult situation according to its unique pattern of strengths and weaknesses. There can be no one best way for families to heal after a child's injury.

The process of recovery does not follow a straight line to the high-est level of recovery the child or adolescent will achieve. There are tremendous cycles of optimism and disappointment as the child progresses or does not. Families observe their children doing amaz-ingly well one day, and having difficulty with some very basic task the next. The child's performance and recovery may seem sporadic and inconsistent.

Developmental Factors

Children's level of functioning represents only a partial attainment of most life skills. The process of development is a process of change. Children learn to accomplish tasks – for example, they acquire voca-tional skills – as they grow towards adulthood. These developmental issues, which are also known as *transitional issues*, refer to the skills a young person needs to move from the dependency of childhood towards adulthood. For the child, completing developmental tasks means acquiring abilities and skills not possessed previously. For these achievements to come about, several basic ingredients are nec-essary. The person has to have an appropriate physiological capabil-ity – for example, the ability to walk. The number of neurons and synapses a child has is another ingredient. These can be looked at as part of the equipment that is necessary to process information from the environment. A brain injury damages neurons and synapses and interrupts ongoing development. This interruption affects not only skills already possessed (or those about to be acquired) but also the ability to acquire new skills and knowledge typical for the child's age. Intellectual development depends on continually learning and retaining more complicated knowledge. If a child's capacity for information processing is lowered, the child's ability to learn will also be lowered. A skill or knowledge deficit may not be detectable until the child needs to use a particular skill. The preparatory work the brain needed to do in order to be able to accomplish the harder jobs of a more mature young person may be only partially completed.

Because children with brain injury are still growing and developing, many of their problems do not show up until later. Life naturally becomes more challenging and complex. Expected and appropriate behaviour for a child varies with age. Certain problems that were not apparent immediately after injury emerge later in development. As the child gets older, the child and the family may be confronted with new issues regularly. This delayed effect is often misunderstood. The injury's implications, for the child's life and capabilities, change as the child grows older. At the same time, the child's awareness of the impact of the injury changes. Adjusting to the effects of injury requires a readjustment at each developmental level.

Children's injuries have a wider variety of causes than adult's. Also, children acquire brain injuries from different causes at different ages. For example, infants and toddlers often sustain a brain injury from physical abuse or a fall. Children between four and twelve are more likely to be victims of falls, sporting accidents, or motor vehicle accidents. The frequency with which children suffer brain injury from motor vehicle accidents increases with age. Adolescents are often involved in high-speed automobile accidents (which are also frequent causes of brain injury in adults). In source and severity, no two children's brain injuries are the same; each has a unique impact on future cognitive development that begins from the point of injury. The injury may be diffuse, or it may be limited to one small site in the brain.

The child's age, temperament, level of cognitive development, and skills prior to the injury together create the unique pattern of the brain injury. Pre-existing health conditions are also a factor. Some differences in outcome are attributable to the child's developmental level at the time of injury. Rapidly developing skills are more vulnerable than firmly established ones. Although a younger child's brain has greater plasticity, the cognitive effects can be just as great as with older children. Brain injury disrupts the development of a range of mental abilities; however, impairment of new learning is the most frequently encountered type of deficit in children and adults.

How disruptive the brain injury is depends on many factors. The earlier in life the brain injury occurs, the less predictable the long-term outcome. On a child reaching adolescence, the effects of an injury sustained in infancy can be quite different from those of a similar injury sustained in late childhood. Physical development (for example, whether puberty is approaching or has been passed) does not help us predict cognitive development. Transitions to the next stage of life can be greatly affected by a brain injury. The long-term consequences of the brain injury may be estimated by means of an IQ test given in the post-acute phase of rehabilitation. However, predictions based solely on clinical judgment may be very different from those drawn from IQ testing.

The Family in Rehabilitation

A child's brain injury poses many problems for the family to solve. If the family has successfully adapted to other crises and has well-developed communication and problem-solving skills, those skills may help them cope. Because the parents have ultimate responsibility for the child, they become service co-ordinators for the long-term care and rehabilitation of their child. Sometimes, especially if there is insurance coverage, they may have the help of a professional case manager. Most children who are hospitalized for brain injury after an accident have no other pre-existing condition such as a neurological, orthopedic, or other ongoing health problem. It is thus unlikely that the parents will have any experience with the special-needs system and its resources.

There are several key factors that influence a family's success in dealing with a child's brain injury. The burden the family was carrying prior to the brain injury can be very important: For example, are there financial or health problems, or is only one parent available? Another factor is the family's ability to adapt and cope; its members may in the past have faced other large problems successfully. Also important is the availability of professional resources – for example, professionals with expertise in pediatric brain injury. There are fewer specialized services for brain-injured children than there are for adults.

Parents need to educate themselves about the long-term effects of brain injury. These may include fatigue, impulsive behaviours, difficulties with social skills, memory loss, irritability, disorganization, shortened attention span, and passivity. Some children may have obvious difficulties with speech, hearing, vision, and/or motor performance. Others may show less visible signs of change but have difficulty concentrating, controlling impulses, or organizing and completing their school work.

Brain injury can traumatize parts of the brain that are central to the behaviours that comprise personality. Cognitive and behaviour changes that result from brain injury seem to be more variable in children than in adults. This must be viewed in the context of a developmental process that is continually changing. Cognitive, maturational, and psychosocial factors interact far more in children than in adults. Changes in personality and social behaviour may mean that young people who were formerly well liked by peers and successful in school may engage in behaviours that disrupt family life, friendships, and schooling. The child or adolescent may not be able to participate in activities that once provided social contact, yet the need to socialize and develop social skills is crucial. Learning to get along with others is a central focus in the lives of children and young people.

A brain injury can lead to troubling changes in behaviour, such as reduced ability to inhibit impulses, irritability, outbursts of anger, impatience, emotional lability or reactivity, and increased aggressiveness. Other behaviours, less noticeable but also troubling, include lack of spontaneity, passivity, decreased initiative and interest, slowness, and fatigue. Lower grades, incidents of disruptive classroom behaviour, complaints by teachers, and feelings of confusion and isolation may be the result of cognitive changes.

Parents need to be able to identify how the brain injury has affected their child's ability to function at home, at school, and in the community. Parents need to be knowledgeable regarding their child's needs and the types of services that will benefit the child. Because they are still developing, many children with brain injury have special needs in common with children who have other health care problems. These could include therapy for deficits in mobility, communication, adaptive skills, and behaviour problems. Some special-education resources and vocational planning may also be needed.

Parents need to develop their observation skills. They can keep a notebook with clinical data on the child – for example, during morning or evening, or when rested or tired, or when participating in solitary and group activities or under various stimuli and distractions. This notebook could also include descriptions of any difficulties with schoolwork. A detailed personal history of the brain-injured young person helps doctors and other professionals understand what may be needed. Parents need to understand that although some changes may be immediately evident (post-injury and upon the child's return home), other changes may not appear until later in the child's recovery. Some signs of difficulty are obvious – for example, a former above-average student performing poorly. Professionals may fail to recognize the change because they did not know the child's previous standard of accomplishment.

A major parental role is advocating for social opportunities, learning options, funding, and other types of resources for their brain-injured child. Parents are also teachers. One important skill they teach their child is how to fit into society and get along with other people. A common problem many parents face is getting their brain-injured child to participate in activities that are good learning opportunities. Parents can present alternatives to the child or adolescent; a young person may find it easier to choose between alternatives than to simply follow instructions. Parents may have to be assertive in order to get reluctant adolescents to join activities in which they can practise important friendship skills; this is often the case when the adolescent perceives some aspects of the activity as less than preferred. The activity may provide much-needed socializing and a chance to behave independently with people other than family members.

Parents can help their child practise explaining to peers why he (she) seems different. Even if the brain injury is not initially detectable, there are times when it is appropriate and therapeutic for brain-injured people to be able to confidently explain their condition to others. They also need to practise emotional self-defence. Children and adolescents are less emotionally defended than adults. They are more vulnerable than adults emotionally, and are disproportionately affected by their social relationships. They experience more anxiety after a brain injury. It may be useful for a member of the rehabilitation team to give a presentation to friends or classmates about brain injury. Someone the same age who has also had an acquired brain injury may help a child or adolescent accept suggestions that would not have been accepted from an adult.

Aunts, uncles, and cousins can provide valuable socializing practice for the injured child. Siblings can also provide needed practice in getting along with other people. This contact can help counteract the loneliness some children feel if their peers move on without them in school and socially. Friendships often do not last when a major change occurs in the personality, physical ability, or behaviour of one of the friends. For many families, religious or spiritual practices can be a support and source of friends. Inviting a child's friends into the home creates opportunities to socialize.

Rebuilding *self-esteem* is very important after a significant injury. Parents know what their child likes and is good at – for example, gardening, computers, arts and crafts, music, cooking, working on bikes or motors. The brain-injured person needs to acquire interests, household responsibilities, and part-time work experiences as soon as possible. These activities can help counter a natural trend toward self-absorption. Children and adolescents are self-centred naturally, and this is a normal developmental issue for them. This self-absorption may be exaggerated by the often lengthy recovery period after a brain injury, and by the resulting isolation from peers. Jobs that the young person can perform for the family – even if they are performed with difficulty and imperfectly – are important. Learning and growing into independence is a process. Parents can reinforce the concept of not quitting even when the job can't be done perfectly.

Over time, a child's brain injury places tremendous strain on the family. Life for most parents is difficult enough. At the time the child was injured, the parents may have feared their child would die. These feelings are among the strongest they will ever experience. Significant emotional disturbance may appear in one or both parents, or the brain-injured child, or the child's siblings. The child or adolescent may require a complex mix of care and yet be less controlled emotionally and behaviourally. This makes providing care more difficult. The other family members may have mixed emotions: they may feel irritable, angry, or sad, and may express these feelings – perhaps inadvertently – to the injured child, or the treatment team, or other family members. The parents of the brain-injured child or adolescent have to cope with a large number of new tasks. Avoiding analysis and problem-solving can make a situation even more difficult. When communication breaks down, consulting a mental health counsellor who is experienced in brain injury may be helpful.

Many professionals consider developing effective household routines to be an important coping strategy. When life has been so disrupted, routines lend predictability and balance. Young people with brain injury may have poor judgment, exaggerated emotional reactions, and problems with impulse control. In these unpredictable and difficult situations, family routines and effective communication provide a stabilizing influence.

Returning to School

The brain-injured child or adolescent is a complex challenge for the school. Sometimes the child will want to change schools rather than return to the original school. On re-entering school, children with brain injury may have physical, sensory, communicative, cognitive/ academic, and social/behavioural problems. Typically, school personnel have little expert or even general knowledge about brain injury.

Schools are a reflection of society, and interest in a particular situation will vary. Some teachers and staff will be prepared to provide the assistance and special attention necessary to develop the child's educational program. Principals and other administrative staff can help create a positive atmosphere at the school, especially if they have some interest or background in special education. However, the staff may choose to define themselves as teachers only of 'average' students with 'average' learning concerns. Schools are funded quite differently from the medical system. Extra attention your child receives may place an additional burden on the school staff.

Parents need to know as much as possible about their child's problem areas in order to explain them to teachers, and to determine whether the program the school offers will be beneficial. Parents have to be assertive and diplomatic, as well as sensitive to the demands facing the school and its staff, if they are to arrange the necessary special services for their brain-injured child. This child is competing for scarce resources, and it is essential for the parents to maintain good working relationships with school staff.

Parents need to know when to request neuropsychological assessment. They should be aware of the types of information the examiner needs regarding the student's strengths and weaknesses. A request for an evaluation needs to be stated in such a way that specific remedial suggestions and techniques will result. The resources and limitations of the school setting need to be considered. Communication/language disorders should be evaluated by a speech/ language pathologist so that the child can receive remedial help – from outside the school, if necessary.

Some of these assessments may have to be paid for by parents or insurers. To plan for a child's needs, and to monitor progress toward independence, it is necessary to understand the child's current state of functioning in the areas noted. Experts can provide more than current status information; they can also help develop strategies for dealing with the child's or adolescent's problems.

An individualized educational program may require that a counsellor or school nurse monitor the child or adolescent while in school. For example, the school nurse may have a bed in her office on which a student can rest if feeling tired. Extra supports might include in-class teaching assistants, access to learning centres outside the regular classroom, and an individualized educational program developed in consultation with special education staff and a school psychologist.

A wide range of educational supports is available, including multimedia resources and word-processing software. Multiple-choice test formats are preferable, and if motivation or self-initiation is low, presenting items in a random, unpredictable order may help maintain the student's interest and involvement. Brain-injured students typically need more structure. However, too much structure may cause brain-injured students to feel that they are being treated below their capabilities and level of maturity.

In terms of responsibility, time, and expense, brain-injured students can place heavy demands on schools. Some schools have few resources and a disproportionate number of students with special needs. These schools may feel they have little to offer.

Private tutoring may help to ensure that the child completes homework assignments. This may also help the child and the parents get along, as homework sessions can be sources of conflict.

Finally, some learning difficulties related to the injury may not be immediately apparent. Needs for special services may not be identified until later stages of the child's recovery, as various brain processes are challenged by different educational tasks and increasingly complex schoolwork. Quite often grandparents, or other persons who see the child less often, will notice a problem before the parents do. Especially relevant are questions such as these: 'Is the child or young person making progress as expected?' 'What would I expect from this child in comparison to others his or her age?' If the child or teen isn't doing what would normally be expected, such as going to parties and dances, and playing sports, this could indicate a problem.

Current diagnostic tools do not reveal all injuries and as the child grows older the learning that needs to take place is more complex. Problems evolve over time. Any reduced speed of work performance and impaired learning ability may become apparent only gradually as the child's chronological age begins to outstrip the progress being made at school. As the child grows older, there should be regular reassessments.

By grade five children may be expected to move to different classrooms for different subjects. The brain-injured young person needs to be able to manage this change. The amount of information the child is expected to know is increasing. Non-brain-injured peers are able to process larger amounts of abstract information. For example, mathematics becomes more abstract, not just rote memorization of facts and calculations. External controls are decreasing, and self-regulation is becoming more expected.

The brain-injured child is socially vulnerable. 'Labelling' – a formal or informal process of identification or description – can be a very negative experience for students when it creates feelings of exclusion. At a very early age, students define themselves in terms of what is considered normal. Being removed from class in an obvious manner to receive learning assistance or special education can result in the student facing rejection or teasing by classmates. Because so many children find it difficult to cope with school, a significant amount of research has been done on this topic. In one study, the researchers found that students with special needs experienced labelling, stigmatization, 'gate-keeping,' bullying, and social rejection.

Brain-injured children tend to get separated from the most desirable social groups at school. As they grow older they may show increasingly awkward social behaviour. When they are separated from their classmates for special education or individual instruction, they lose opportunities to socialize. They need more opportunities to be with children their own age. These situations need to be seen as opportunities to coach the child on socially acceptable behaviour.

The school's social environment provides most of the opportunities for social learning. Social needs and peer interactions are extremely important for a child or adolescent. Making new friends and dealing with peer rejection is often more difficult after a brain injury.

The complexity of social interaction increases between elementary school and junior and senior high. There are more shades of grey. The concept of *commitment* becomes more important, and there are degrees of relationship. Friendships involve more complex knowledge – for example, of families and sexual behaviour. Parents need to ask questions such as these: 'What isolates them from the group?' 'Is their voice too loud?' 'Do they crowd others?' (If a group of socially desirable peers want to talk privately, the brain-injured person must know to gracefully move on without hard feelings, leaving room for another social contact at another time). 'Are they touching others or hugging inappropriately?' 'Are they too quiet, and would assertiveness training help?' 'Can they manage their anger?' Difficulties communicating emotions and needs, and recognizing one's own emotions, and thinking before acting are all ongoing, coachable issues. A young person who is unable to confide that he or she is experiencing difficulty with peers is more likely to act inappropriately and develop behaviour problems. Not being included socially with the friends of one's choice creates stress and can compel teens to associate with persons who have social problems themselves. Yet the brain-injured young person may not understand the implications of being friends with teens who, for example, are often 'in trouble.'

In summary, students with special needs manage their disabilities in school in a number of positive and negative ways. Staying in school and completing as much education as possible, even though it may be very difficult, enhances a person's chances of achieving independence and having more choices in life.

Safety Issues

It is natural for the parents of a brain-injured child to be very concerned about safety. They may need to feel they have some control, especially if they have been through a harrowing experience in which they feared their child might die. However, the parents' protective behaviour may create conflict with their child, who may be going through the natural developmental phase of separating from the parents and wanting to do new, perhaps risky, activities under reduced parental supervision.

There are many issues for the teen. Is he or she able to drive safely? Professional driving evaluators can assist in determining this. Attention problems, impulsivity, impaired judgment, and uncontrolled outbursts of anger could make driving too risky. The brain-injured adolescent will be acquiring some life skills for the first time. Learning a new skill *after* a brain injury can be more difficult than relearning a well practised, previously learned skill. Driving a car, for example, is an overlearned skill that most adults do almost unconsciously. If the component abilities are still intact, an adult who has many years of driving experience may be able to resume driving after a series of lessons. However, a young person with similar injury may need many more hours of instruction to drive competently.

Professionals who have worked with brain injury survivors have observed that individuals often received their injury on a Friday night or after having used alcohol or other drugs. Research studies have demonstrated an association between brain injury and substance abuse. Many young teens have social opportunities to use alcohol and drugs, and these may have strong appeal. Adolescence is a stressful time of life, so it is not difficult to understand the appeal of alcohol or drugs.

Alcohol may dull the pain of anxiety, depression, or injured self-esteem. Family members may also use alcohol to help cope with painful feelings. The young person may be drawn to alcohol or drugs as a means of escaping awareness of the disability. Other methods for responding to these normal feelings must be found.

Alcohol is not recommended for a brain-injured person because the injury itself can change and amplify the characteristic effects of alcohol. Some brain injury survivors are prescribed pain and anticonvulsant medications, and these may not be compatible with alcohol use. Brain injury may limit a person's ability to inhibit impulses and may negatively affect a person's judgment. Drinking alcohol reduces a person's ability to monitor the consequences of behaviour, just as brain injury itself does. Impaired judgment puts the young person at risk for another accident, and for other negative consequences.

The child or adolescent needs physical exercise and should not withdraw from all fitness activities. Many safe and healthy fitness options are available. Contact sports are not recommended because of the risk of reinjuring the brain: the effects of more than one brain injury can be cumulative.

Attention problems make operating power tools potentially dangerous, especially since a brain-injured person's ability to perform complex tasks is reduced during times of fatigue. Is the brain-injured child aware that his or her abilities are affected by fatigue? Such awareness requires some self-monitoring ability, which in turn depends on the specific nature of the brain injury. Especially for younger children, parents should closely monitor climbing activity. This is wise advice whether the child has a brain injury or not. Potentially dangerous behaviour needs to be reviewed very carefully with young brain-injured people, even though they may not fully appreciate the need for this review. The information   is sometimes more acceptable coming from persons other than the parents.

Case Study

The following case illustrates the complex issues families face when their teenager acquires a brain injury.

Nicole was a very attractive seventeen-year-old girl who received a brain injury in a motor vehicle accident when she was sixteen. Her brain injury was considered moderate in severity, with a Glasgow Coma Scale rating of 9. She was the youngest of four children. Her three older siblings had left home, and her father's work regularly kept him away from home on week-long business trips. After returning home from hospital, she complained of painful headaches, balance problems, sleep problems, and fatigue. She missed half of one year of school and returned part-time, taking one course. Prior to her accident she had a history of learning problems, and she had received some special learning assistance while in elementary school. One year after her injury, her problems included a visual memory deficit (especially after some time had elapsed since she had seen the object to be remembered), fatigue, headaches, and difficulty concentrating. Some personality changes had been reported by Nicole's parents. Previously Nicole had been shy and withdrawn; now she was louder and more socially forward. She had frequent angry outbursts and was more emotionally explosive. These outbursts had become less frequent in the year since her brain injury, but they were still occurring on a daily basis. She complained that her parents were treating her like they did when she was thirteen. She had difficulty appreciating another person's point of view. She found it extremely difficult to tolerate restrictions on her freedom, and was very sensitive to any criticism of her behaviour. She also did not see any reason why she should not resume driving. Her parents' concerns centred on her more outward social behaviour, on the possible risks this behaviour exposed her to, on her outbursts of anger, and on her inability to appreciate their perspective and feelings. As a result, they did not feel she was ready to resume driving.

11. Couple Issues After Brain Injury*

Patrick Hirschi, MSW, RSW
Claudia Berwald, MSW, RSW
Rick Brown, MSW, RSW

You Are All Survivors

Brain injury is not an isolated incident in one person's life. It's a life-transforming event that affects not only the injured person, but that person's family, friends, and workmates. *Everyone* is a survivor. Possibly, the most profound impact is on the spousal union. This impact varies in nature and intensity, depending on where the two people are in their life as a partnership, but it is always powerful. Young couples without children are spared some of the challenges that couples with young children must face. Couples whose children have left home face some different issues as well.

The relationship that the two partners have with each other changes, as do family roles and responsibilities. At least for a time, the injured survivor becomes dependent on his or her partner for a

*Much of this chapter was adapted from *The Survivors* video and discussion guide series, written by David Pare and Patrick Hirschi and published in 1995 by the Glenrose Rehabilitation Hospital, Edmonton, Alberta.

This series was produced as part of the *Distance Education and Support Groups for Family Caregivers of Brain Injury Survivors* project.

Principal investigator: Rick Brown

Project team members: Claudia Berwald, Rosalyn Delehanty, Patrick Hirschi, Harry Miller, and Kerrie Pain variety of things previously taken for granted. Interpersonal communication becomes an incredible challenge for couples as they struggle to cope with the many changes that follow a brain injury. Old patterns of communicating often do not work as well as before the injury.

With all these changes come the intense feelings that accompany any loss – shock, denial, anger, and depression. However, most survivors find ways to cope, using their own inner resources or reaching out to others; they manage to move on and find some new, positive meaning in their lives. In this chapter we will be exploring the complex and difficult couple issues that follow a brain injury.

Case Example

Mary and Bill had just gotten married and were on their honeymoon out of province when they were involved in a car collision. Mary sustained an extremely severe traumatic brain injury. Her post-traumatic amnesia would persist for over six months. Her treatment in an acute-care hospital took over two months, after which she went directly to an in-patient brain injury program at a rehabilitation hospital for another three-and-a-half months of intensive therapy. Mary had to relearn how to walk, dress, eat, and speak. Thus began her long journey of recovery.

As a direct result of the accident, the couple's life together took an abrupt turn. Their future plans had to be placed on hold. Just before the accident, Mary had completed the third year of a four-year nursing degree. Bill was working as a tradesman but had plans to go on in school to become a minister. The couple, by marrying, had committed themselves to spending their lives together, and the marriage had been witnessed by family and friends.

After Mary returned home from the rehabilitation hospital, she still needed supervision to ensure her safety. To that end, Bill quit his job and took on the responsibility of providing care for his wife. He also had to take on other responsibilities, such as taking care of the house and the family finances. Mary's gradual return to more independence would take several years; gradually, Bill would be able to resume his work. Their extended families became much more involved in their lives after the accident, and this created tensions. Bill and Mary sought couple counselling to deal with these. Both also reached out separately for support: Bill attended a caregiver out-patient group, while Mary attended a support group for people with brain injury. This support was valuable to both Mary and Bill, as it helped them sort out their own feelings about the multiple psycho-social issues brought to the fore by Mary's injury.

As Mary slowly developed more insight into her changed abilities and realized that she would not be able to resume her schooling, she began to struggle with depression. To help her feel better about herself and her future, both she and Bill sought out community resources to help her fill her day with volunteer programs, recreational activities, and opportunities to take courses.

Bill had to revise many of his plans for his own future, and that of his marriage, in the light of the many barriers now preventing him from returning to school. For example, he and Mary considered the challenges involved in becoming parents, and sought out information about the special difficulties they might face as parents. Five years after the accident, their life has changed in ways that no one could have predicted. However, by working out their own feelings about the accident, and by working on their own communications as a couple, Mary and Bill have been able to confront these unexpected challenges. Now they have settled their litigation, and bought a home, and have a beautiful daughter, and they are looking forward to their future as a family.

Managing Changes to Roles and Relationships

Non-injured spouses typically experience an altogether different set of role changes than the injured survivor. The changes may be obvi-ous from the outset, as the non-injured spouse quickly takes on the role of 'chauffeur' or 'nurse' in daily visits to the hospital. The same spouse may take over the role of family breadwinner, or of 'parent' to the injured partner. A brain injury may lead to the non-injured spouse taking on management of finances, or home maintenance, or correspondence with friends and extended family. With the change of duties comes a change of identity: our work tends to play a large part in defining who we are. Sometimes the experience of taking on new tasks is overwhelming, and the need for support becomes critical. At other times the non-injured spouse discovers previously hidden strengths and qualities. Whichever is the case, brain injury calls on all survivors to find new parts of themselves as they adjust to the changes in their lives.

Children of an injured survivor may be deeply troubled by the sudden helplessness of a parent who was once a model of competence and strength. For the uninjured parent, parenting then becomes a tremendous challenge, with limited opportunities to share in successes, failures, and responsibilities. Children may react in a variety of ways depending on their age, their level of maturity, and their communication skills. They require special support to avoid developing feelings of being 'forgotten,' as much of the attention must now be focused on the injured survivor. This is where the support of the extended family becomes critical to help fill the void.

Uninjured spouses may feel a yearning to share their worries and hopes with the injured partner, only to find that the communication channels are clogged. While brain injury sometimes brings families and couples closer, it also creates a tremendous strain on relationships, as survivors struggle to adapt to a changed world.

Communication and parenting are not the only issues couples have to face. Many injured survivors, be they female or male, lose their 'libido,' or sex drive. Less often, sex drive increases dramatically in the injured survivor. Both scenarios are usually very confusing and distressful for both the non-injured spouse and injured survivors, at a time when patience and trust are at a premium.

Many *non-injured* spouses also experience a dramatic reduction in their sex drive. This results from fatigue, worry, and increased responsibility, and also from the disheartening feeling that they are living and sleeping with a 'stranger.' Couples really need to take the time to get to know each other again – to learn again how to enjoy touching and cuddling, and to seek counselling if difficulties with intimacy and sexuality persist. At the same time, non-injured spouses often wrestle with feelings of guilt that arise from their yearning for more personal space. This yearning is sometimes mixed with a powerful need to take over and do almost everything for the injured survivor. Finding the right mix takes patience, understanding, and a willingness to talk and listen.

Balancing Dependence and Independence

For the non-injured spouse, the urge to regain some personal freedom is usually coupled with a fear of letting go – a fear that comes from a deep caring, and from concern that the injured survivor might become injured again or die. All of us, whether we have been injured or not, rely on others for some of our needs. However, in the first several months after a brain injury, injured survivors usually become almost totally dependent. The non-injured spouse is thus called on to fill a role that may be quite unfamiliar. This is a dramatic change in circumstances for everyone involved. The needs of the injured survivor may be all-consuming. Someone who was once a partner, a peer, or a parent may be more like an infant again, bringing to the relationship all of the demands of an earlier, more childlike stage of life. Everything takes longer; time is at a premium, so that time for oneself will sometimes seem nonexistent. Time for relationships – with friends or with other family members – may be equally rare. Adding to this extra pressure is the fact that the non-injured spouse often receives less material and emotional support from the injured survivor. As a result, the non-injured spouse often relies more heavily on others for help in meeting these needs.

Many non-injured spouses say they're torn between the need to protect the survivor and the need to push the survivor toward greater independence. At the same time, the personal needs of the non-injured spouse may begin to resurface. After a long period of selflessness, he or she may yearn for more space and time. Feelings of guilt often arise from this. Mixed with the other powerful feelings brought on by brain injury, the struggle for balance makes for an emotional roller coaster.

Spouses often report feeling unsure about their own judgment of what is best for the injured survivor. They question their motives: Are they holding the injured survivor back without good cause? Are they pushing the survivor too hard? The difference between the spouse's view and that of the injured survivor can make for considerable confusion. The only solution is good communication.

Communication Challenges

It's a challenge to keep the lines of communication open after a brain injury. Everyone involved feels vulnerable in the wake of such a trauma, which thoroughly upsets the balance of life. Physical limitations and changes in thinking patterns may block the clear exchange of messages. And the stress of the new life situation adds to the likelihood of derailed communication. Keeping the lines of communication open is critical to maintaining supportive relationships after a brain injury. In households hampered by unshared thoughts and feelings, the weight of unspoken words can be crippling. This is why it's important to be aware of the many obstacles to clear and honest dialogue that may arise in the wake of a brain injury.

For both the spouses and injured survivors, communicating in the context of these changes to physical abilities and cognitive patterns is like playing a board game with a revised set of rules: you're working towards the same purpose, but the obstacles are different. A message sent may not be clearly received. The result, for both spouse and injured survivor, is often intense frustration and misunderstanding. There is the risk of falling back on old assumptions about the injured survivor's abilities, values, interests, and points of view, only to discover unexpected misunderstandings or disagreements.

Changes in cognitive abilities are another common source of communication breakdown. Injured survivors are often unaware of their own cognitive deficits. For example, they may think their memory is fine, even as they forget the topic of a conversation in mid-sentence. This gap between injured survivors' self-perceptions and the perceptions of others often leads to frustration and misunderstanding. But it isn't only the injured survivors who change in the aftermath of brain injury. Parents, partners, children, and others close to the injured survivor typically find themselves wearing many new hats, assuming unfamiliar roles, and becoming burdened by extra responsibilities. Throughout all this, the injured survivor may not be able to provide as much emotional support as the spouse feels he or she needs. The common feelings of resentment, anger, and guilt that arise often stand in the way of open and clear communication.

For all survivors, stress is another factor that inevitably affects communication and the harmony of relationships. When people are anxious, or tired, or otherwise struggling with massive changes in their lives, it's natural for friction to arise – brain injury or no brain injury.

For couples, the process starts with a fundamental examination of the relationship. Can we do this together? Are we able and willing to live with the massive changes we face as a partnership? When couples stay together even though these questions are unresolved, the issue hovers over them, and makes it difficult to move ahead in life.

Even with the resolve to make a go of it, the communication challenges posed by brain injury call for much learning and adaptation by everyone involved. Non-injured spouses who succeed – and many do – come to identify areas of strength and weakness; they learn to avoid exchanges that will almost certainly lead to misunderstanding, and to rely on the modes of communication that are most likely to succeed.

Coping with Loss

Survivors of brain injury, as well as their spouses, are often told that no two injuries are alike. This is with good reason. The experience of brain injury varies from person to person, often in dramatic and unexpected ways. However, one factor is common to all people affected by brain injury – *the experience of loss*. After a brain injury, we naturally tend to place a great deal of our attention on what has been taken from the injured survivor. But spouses also experience a wide range of losses. They, too, may long for the relationship they once had with their partner. And they must cope with drastic changes in lifestyle that usually involve an increase in personal responsibilities and a decrease in mobility and flexibility. For entire families, brain injury may mean the loss of connection to friends, and to a whole range of activities in the outside world. These changes are coupled with powerful feelings that rise up over and over again.

If you are a non-injured spouse you may be so focused on the changes in the injured survivor that you fail to notice changes in yourself. But you are also a survivor, and your own world has been altered – often in very dramatic ways. Non-injured spouses, no less than injured ones, must adapt to major lifestyle and relationship changes, and to the sense of loss that goes with them.

After the initial shock, the grieving begins for both the injured survivor and the spouses. Grieving takes many forms, from outrage and denial, to profound sadness and despair. There is often a sense of profound injustice, that life has lost all meaning. Most survivors say they have experienced each of these feelings at different times, and that they continue to experience them – though perhaps not so intensely – long after the initial injury.

A great loss brings a sense of bewilderment to life. It's as though the world has been turned upside down, so that the pieces all fall in unexpected places. It's difficult to make sense of that new world, in which we have been robbed of something precious. It's hard to know where to place our trust, hard to plan for a future that is clouded with uncertainty.

For some survivors, coping with the losses that follow brain injury can be a lonely process. Brain injury brings some families together, but it may also prompt family members to draw back, out of their own fear and discomfort around the deep feelings surrounding brain injury. Others who are not directly involved may have difficulty relating to the experience of survivors, and trouble offering the support they would like to.

Whatever their approach to coping, all survivors of brain injury describe a drawn-out process of reorienting to their situation, readjusting to their new life. Facing these changes takes courage. Often the determination to move forward comes with a feeling of hope that shines like a beacon at the end of a dark tunnel. With time, what seemed bewildering begins to make sense. The world takes on a new meaning. It's a profound process – a rediscovery of life.

Taking Stock and Reaching Out

Brain injury poses new limitations, but also new possibilities. Each day, you rise to meet a unique set of challenges. In your own way, you have already begun to develop many new coping skills. As 'survivors,' and as a couple, you have much to share, much to learn, and much to give. Reaching out to others is not always easy in the middle of the crisis of brain injury. It takes courage to trust others, and to face feelings that are often very painful. And yet most of the hundreds of survivors of brain injury we have worked with say that their greatest comfort comes from sharing their experience with family, friends, and other survivors.

Another part of the task of adjusting to brain injury is to discover just what you need to do to take care of yourself, and how to continue to care for the ones you love during trying times. There is no right or wrong way to cope. Some survivors say they need to share their feelings with others regularly, while others put a priority on carving out some personal space for themselves. A good cry is sometimes a great release; but others report that humour and laughter do the job just as well. Many survivors seem to benefit from focusing on solutions rather than problems.

You will learn what works for you by paying attention to how you feel, to how your approach helps you and your loved ones get through each day. You may find that your own approach to coping has changed since the brain injury. Or perhaps you have a way of dealing with hard times that you fall back on over and over again. Whatever your approach to coping, it's useful to recognize it and name it. If you do, you can cope effectively in times of need.

Finding New Meaning in Life

Brain injury asks survivors to make a big shift – to act, think, and feel differently. To succeed in the wake of the injury is to open up to new possibilities and new ways of being. For couples, this difference may provoke a crisis that must be addressed before they can move on. They may feel like strangers to each other. Or their relationship may have become unbalanced, with one partner becoming in some ways a helpless child, and the other an all-powerful and responsible parent.

Although relationship issues may hold up the process of moving on after brain injury, that process isn't solved by deciding to stay or deciding to leave. Like anyone else, survivors of brain injury are faced with a lifelong project: the task of coping with the trials that life sets. Non-injured spouses often discover the need for personal space and private time, to counterbalance lives that have become filled with caregiving responsibilities. Exercise or hobby classes, solo walks, social outings, quiet times on the living room couch with a good book – there is no end to the ways that spouses can take time out from their duties and responsibilities.

Brain Injury Is What You Make of It

Because of the dramatic changes that brain injury brings to peoples' lives, its impact goes far beyond surface appearances. Survivors and their spouses often change their lifestyle, develop new circles of friends, reconnect with family members, and revise their future plans. More often than not, they also report a profound rethinking of their lives, a new outlook that's evident in the way they look at everything around them.

In our work with families and couples, we've found that those who adjust most successfully learn at some stage to look on the positive side of their experience ... to identify the welcome changes introduced into their lives as a result of the injury. This glimpse of the bright side can make coping a lot easier when life seems overwhelming. Depending on where you are at in your adjustment to brain injury, you may or may not have experienced this change in outlook. It's a revisioning of your life that unfolds naturally, but also one that can be nurtured and developed by focusing on the positive aspects of your new life context.

12. Brain Injury and the Family System

Carroll O. David, MSSW

Traumatic brain injury changes the survivor's view of both the self and the world. The effects on the family are equally great. For both the survivor and the family, recovery is a long process that lasts for years – and for many, a lifetime.

More often than not, survivors will deny the effects the injury is having on their behaviour, thus making it difficult for the family to respond in helpful ways.

Over time, both the family and the survivor can change their expectations to fit what is possible; they can find new ways to relate, and learn how to make room for the needs of everyone involved. But this task is neither easy nor simple. There are no easy solutions or quick fixes.

The Family as a System

When a part of our body is injured, our muscles recoil; our blood clots; antibodies are produced in our bloodstream; and pain reminds us to protect the injured part. It is clear how the different parts of our body work together. Within a family, injury to one member affects all other members, and just as our body reacts to physical injury, the individuals respond as a unit. The family's activities during this crisis may seem jumbled to an outsider, but if we look closely we can see that the family's response is much more organized than it first seems. Usual activities are put on hold, plans are changed, needs and

Grandfather Grandmother			Grandfather Grandmother		
Father			Mother		
		Child			
		Child			
		Child			

FIGURE 12.1 'Typical' Family Structure (straight lines represent generational boundaries).

decisions are put off, responsibilities are divided, and working together is given priority. The family's level of energy increases as it mobilizes resources to meet the emergency.

The family does its job of nurturing, protecting, and socializing its members through subsystems. A *subsystem* is any unit smaller than the whole family group. The smallest unit is the individual. Other subsystems are husband/wife, father/mother, mother/child, father/child, and siblings. Subsystems are formed by functions, such as parenting; by generation, such as brothers and sisters; or by gender, such as mother/daughter or father/son. There are boundaries around each subsystem that define the rules for who its members are, and who participates and how. When a mother tells an older son that he is not a younger son's parent, and that *she* will correct the younger son if necessary, she is clearly marking the boundaries between the parental and sibling subsystems.

How a family is organized may be seen in other ways. A father who holds back from disciplining a child, though he is quite capable of doing so, is encouraging the mother to act as the parent in charge. A mother who holds strong opinions may avoid expressing those opinions, thus encouraging the father to speak for the whole family. A child may be given authority over younger siblings in the parents' absence, and give up that role when the parents return. A father who is overly involved in outside activities may shift the burden of parenting to the mother. Thus, all individuals in the family learn to back one another up, and give one another approval and support. They also learn to stress one another in open and not so open ways.

It is important to realize that what stresses one part stresses the whole, and that what stresses the whole stresses each of its parts. If mother is ill, father may have to do double-duty, and the children may have to accept increased responsibilities. If there are financial problems, mother may have to go to work, and older siblings may have to help supervise younger ones. A family works best when it has the flexibility to change roles to fit changing circumstances.

Membership and Development

There is always stress when events require the family to adjust in ways to which is not accustomed. Changes in *family membership*, like the birth of a child, or a death in the family, or a divorce, result in changes that affect how the family operates, both as a whole and within each of its subsystems. There are also *developmental* changes – for example, a child starting school, or entering adolescence, or the retirement of one or both parents. With age, adults in the family also change developmentally. Stress often increases when families are unable to change with changing circumstances – for example, when parents treat adolescents according to rules that worked when they were younger; or when a single parent tries to retain the same style of behaviour as when both parents were present; or when a couple fails to renegotiate their relationship after the last child leaves home.

Membership and developmental changes do not usually become a crisis; that being said, they are important landmarks in family life – that is, times when change is necessary.

With brain injury *it is always a crisis for the family*. A family can prepare for raising children, moving, changing jobs, or adjusting to a divorce; with brain injury, there is no warning and the impact is sudden. The disruptions in daily routines – in who does what, and how and when – are immediate and urgent. Roles involving transportation, schedules, meal times, social commitments, housekeeping, finances, and communicating with health care providers, all must be addressed at a time the family is very anxious about the survivor. The family is in a state of constant vigilance, and its members are concentrating intensely. Who will sit with the survivor? Who will

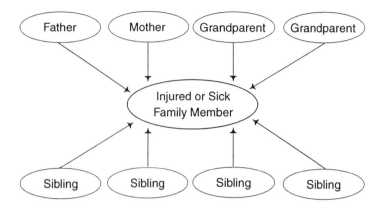

FIGURE 12.2 Family in Crisis

speak for the family? What areas of family life must be changed, delayed, or abandoned? All these questions must be answered.

Reintegrating the Survivor in the Family

When a brain injury survivor returns home, it is often not clear what it means in terms of changes in family membership. If the survivor is reintroduced to his or her pre-injury role, this uncertainty increases, since cognitive and behavioural deficits will interfere with the performance of previous roles. Thus, a student may not be able to function in school, or perform daily tasks, or be competitively employed, or remember daily events.

The family is confronted with a 'new member' as well as the loss of the survivor's ability to function as in the past. The normal course of grieving, which all families experience, is taking place while the family is trying to bring the changed survivor back into the family in a workable way. The survivor must also adjust to the ways in which he or she and the family have changed. Instant adjustment is not possible. The family members and the survivor will need plenty of time to get to know one another in new and different ways. The process takes months, and sometimes years.

As improvement continues beyond the early stages, it often seems to the family that relief is in sight; after all, the survivor can now talk, walk, and ask for things. When the survivor returns home, as most eventually do, the problem becomes not someone who must learn to feed himself or move a limb, but someone who gets lost, repeats himself or herself, and is negative, demanding, paranoid, frightened, self-centred, and unmotivated. This is far more stressful for the family than nursing the survivor to physical recovery. In this situation parents may find themselves blaming each other; spouses may feel dominated by the needs of the injured spouse; siblings may feel short-changed; and extended family, who have only a partial grasp of the situation, may be too quick to criticize. The adjustment process, which during this time can be very difficult, will be faster if family members are active in educating themselves and the extended family about brain injury, and if they openly discuss the impact that brain injury has on each person. Family meetings to address these issues allow each member to know what others are thinking and feeling. Members of the extended family who are poorly informed can be included in these gatherings. Each person can be asked to speak, including the children. It is helpful for primary caregivers to say directly and out loud: 'I want your support. I need your help.' Some creative families publish newsletters periodically updating all members of the family.

Spouses, parents, and siblings often will not express strong feelings about their situation, out of guilt, or for fear it would suggest they are not coping well. They may act in ways which suggest that only the survivor has the right to complain. This is unfortunate, since it encourages the family to focus on the survivor's disability, and discourages communication and decision making about other family matters. It may also lead to overprotectiveness toward survivors, who may then become excessively dependent, which only add stress to an already stressful situation. Since many families view the survivor as fragile and/or incompetent, they often need support in requiring the survivor to accommodate to the family's reality. Health care providers who are knowledgeable about brain injury can help the family be clear and direct about what they can and cannot realistically expect from the survivor. Firmness about what is expected provides limits that survivors are not able to set for themselves. When the family clearly and firmly communicates what it expects, its members gain a sense of empowerment, the survivor is encouraged to work toward more functional behaviour. Saying, 'I want you to shower, brush your teeth, and make your bed. When you are done, then you may have breakfast,' is far better than telling the survivor during breakfast, 'Don't you think you should shower and make your bed?' An approach based on the idea that if the rewards come first, the survivor can be seduced into complying, encourages the survivor to be seductive rather than self-disciplined.

Coping Styles

Families who are *extremely close* emotionally can be especially vulnerable, since the absence of clearly defined roles and expectations tends to increase the survivor's confusion about what is expected. In this style of coping, the family is so intimately involved in every aspect of the survivor's functioning that messages regarding who does what, and how and when, are not always clear, and independent thinking and acting is overlooked. Making decisions for those who are able to do it themselves inhibits self-mastery. Often, very close-knit families prize 'belongingness' over self-mastery. The family members, being strongly committed to ensuring belongingness, may turn mostly to one another, and by-pass the support that can be gained through involvement in the community. This discourages friendships, which are important to both the survivor and the family.

On the other hand, families that are *emotionally distant*, may be poorly informed about problems that various members are experiencing. As a result, the survivor may lose out on valuable support. Perhaps the family is unaware that an adolescent is skipping school. An emotionally distant family may allow the survivor to be exposed to situations with which he or she is unable to cope, out of an unwillingness to interfere with the survivor's 'independence.'

Families who become aware of their own coping styles can alter these styles. Thus emotionally close-knit families can create emotional distance to encourage learning, and emotionally distant families can move closer to provide support. Most of us have coping styles that fall somewhere between these two, so that we are close about some things and distant about others.

Extended Family

Relatives, especially grandparents, may assume functions usually performed by members of the nuclear family, often in partnership with an uninjured spouse. This may weaken subsystem boundaries – that is, parents or spouses may re-establish dependency on their families of origin. 'Who has responsibility for what?' is a far more important question than 'Who is conventionally or traditionally expected to have that responsibility?'

THE K FAMILY

Joe is twenty-five years old and was injured when a delivery truck ran a stop sign and broadsided his car. He was married six months before his injury, to Connie, who is twenty years old. Connie was two months pregnant at the time Joe was injured. Joe had been working as an apprentice in a stock brokerage firm. He has a college degree in business and excelled as a student. He was highly regarded at work for his good judgment and ability to learn quickly. Following post-acute rehabilitation, Joe had problems with his memory, was easily confused (particularly when confronted with a change in routine), and had some difficulty with his balance. Joe's parents are on the verge of retirement and have been making more and more of the decisions regarding his care. Connie felt over-whelmed, particularly several months after his injury after it was clear that Joe still had difficulties. Later she became involved in his rehabilitation and increasingly interested in having something to say about his care and treatment. When Connie complained to several health care workers that her in-laws were taking charge of 'most everything,' the health care providers empathized with her against her 'intrusive' in-laws. This increased the tension between the young wife and the survivor's parents. Had Connie been encouraged to speak directly to Joe's parents about her fears of being 'displaced,' and praised for showing strength in allowing her in-laws to be supportive in extraordinary circumstances, the possibility of mutual support would have increased. It is not 'abnormal' for the parents to become involved under these circumstances.

Children

When a parent is injured, older children may be asked to help care for younger siblings. Older adolescents may be asked to join the uninjured parent in making difficult decisions, and this may result in a complete role reversal in relation to the injured parent. Younger children may be expected to adjust to an older sibling, who now has greater authority than before. Too typically, children are expected to adjust with little attention to what they are experiencing, and often with limited information. Children seeing a parent badly hurt, and the other parent grief-stricken and struggling with a wide range of pressing concerns, will often not ask for information or talk about their own worries, for fear of adding to the parent's burden.

THE S FAMILY

Tim was injured the year following high school graduation. As a student he was above average, socially popular, and a very good amateur musician. At the time of the injury he was pursuing a career as a welder. This was disappointing to his family, who had hoped he would go on to university. Tim has two sisters, one younger and one older, and a brother who is the oldest child and who left home prior to Tim's accident. The accident involved one vehicle, with Tim as the driver. His older sister was a passenger and was also injured, though she was not brain injured. Tim had been drinking when the accident occurred. Following a lengthy period of in-patient rehabilitation, Tim was placed in a group home, and over the next year his behaviour deteriorated steadily. His family described how he drank a six-pack of beer daily, chain-smoked, wandered the streets, and was unemployed. His family intervened and had him placed in a highly structured, behaviourally oriented rehabilitation centre. During this time he and his family, which included his younger sister, age fifteen, his older sister, and both his parents, met with a family therapist. The parents talked at great length about the stresses and difficulties they had encountered during Tim's recovery, and his sister's, and about their efforts to secure 'proper placement for Tim.' Both parents and the older sister spoke freely. The therapist noticed that the youngest sister remained very quiet throughout the session. He asked what she did to help her parents during this prolonged crisis. Her reply: 'Nothing. Mom and Dad took care of everything.' Gently challenging her, the therapist asked how that could be, since she was obviously a very competent and active member of the family. She burst into tears, explaining that she made sure she did not burden her family with any of her concerns, whether it was homework or her friends. After the meeting the father, in tears, said, 'I had no idea she was hurting so much. How did we not see that?'

But at the same time, children who do speak up or complain may not be 'heard' because the needs of the survivor come first. Non-injured adults in the family can play a vital role in reaching out to children, not only by giving them 'permission' to talk about their concerns and ask questions, but also by acknowledging them when they do speak up. It is important to encourage very young children to express their thoughts and feelings, and to give them information. Though they may only understand a small part, doing so sends a powerful message that important adults have an interest in their experiences.

Spouses

With the emphasis our culture places on individual self-reliance, the non-injured spouse faces unique stresses. He or she not only must contend with the loss of a partner, but must also become family spokesperson, sole decision maker, and advocate on behalf of the survivor. The same person must assume single parenthood, educate and negotiate with the extended family, address financial issues, be a companion and support to the injured spouse, and negotiate with lawyers and insurance carriers. Further, the non-injured spouse often must assume a caregiving role with the survivor – a role no one expects to have in a marriage.

THE G COUPLE

Dr G, fifty-five years old, a veterinarian and accomplished eques-trian, was injured when he was kicked by a horse he was training. He was in a coma for several weeks, and after several months of rehabilitation went to live with his wife of twenty-five years. They had three grown sons, all married. Mrs G worked diligently as a caretaker, helping him dress, supervising his activities, and attempt-ing to deal with his impulsiveness and increasingly violent temper. Her approach was to 'give in' in the belief that he would 'come to his senses on his own.' On more than one occasion he slipped out of the house without her being aware, and was returned by the police or by friends who recognized him. He was well known in the small com-munity where they lived. On each occasion he was furious that 'they' were interfering with his freedom, and threatened to sue and file charges. When his wife explained that they were simply trying to help, he accused her of being 'on their side,' and said he could no longer trust her, and refused thereafter to sleep in their bedroom. The more she attempted to 'help,' the more agitated he became, in one instance turning the dining room table over and threatening to throw her out of the house bodily. She often called their adult son, who would come over and try to calm his father. She and her son agreed that Dr G was not only not improving, he was getting worse, and that it was not an option for him to continue staying at home. It had been her hope that Dr G could continue his veterinary practice, especially since they had borrowed a large sum of money prior to his injury and were financially strained.

During a five-year stay as an in-patient in a rehabilitation centre, Dr G improved greatly. He was visited often by his wife. She found that she still could not communicate satisfactorily with him, in spite of his improvement. Dr G remained suspicious that she was seeing another man, and that that was why she had him in rehabilitation. Marital counselling was started, and though their relationship improved for a brief time, it became increasingly clear that Mrs G had little hope for re-establishing the marriage. With great courage, and with support from other spouses who had had similar experi-ences, she filed for divorce. Dr G's family was critical of her decision, as were some of her children, who accused her of abandoning 'our father.' Dr G remained bitter for several months but gradually was able to accept the inevitable. With much support from his children, he eventually returned to his home community, where he met another woman, whom he later married, and resumed his veterinary practice part time.

The G family's experience illustrates that brain injury to a spouse has a dramatic effect on the marriage. Often the changes cannot be corrected. Non-injured spouses who decide to end the marriage are often severely criticized by their children and in-laws and by the extended family. 'Outside' support from health care providers, ministers, friends, family physicians or therapists is crucial in implementing what is usually a very courageous and painful step.

Many support groups are good at providing information on brain injury and behavioural problems in general, but do not deal effectively with the unique needs of spouses. Many spouses relate that groups that are made up of non-injured spouses, and that focus on the specific stresses and needs of spouses, are far more helpful.

Divorced Parents

Not infrequently, the parents of a survivor are separated or divorced. In such situations, unresolved marital issues from the past become significant. In any family, parents compromise their parenting role when they involve children in marital conflicts. Divorced or separated parents should realize that talking negatively about the other parent to the survivor is asking the survivor to take sides. The survivor either plays one parent against the other, or must be very careful not to alienate either parent. Differences regarding custody, guardianship, and medical decisions can be mediated by third parties without involving the survivor.

Identity

Brain injury has an emotional impact on families that may result in changes in how family members interact with one another. For example, a mother who was very close to her overachieving son agreed with her son that his father was insensitive and controlling. Now she is faced with an injured son and a deeply saddened father who needs her support. The father, who prior to the injury saw her as spoiling their son, is now faced with a wife who is grief-stricken and depressed. The parents need each other's support, but they will not have it unless they talk about the issue openly. Here, previous alliances – however workable or unworkable – have shifted, and this requires attention.

Family as Advocate

In the acute recovery phase, families are often left to fend for themselves. If the survivor is in a post-acute rehabilitation setting, usually it is only when the family's involvement is perceived as disruptive that family issues are taken into account. Sometimes the family is labelled a 'problem,' which creates tension in their relationship with health providers. Some families, though they want to criticize, will not do so for fear of losing the health provider's support. A lack of information almost always aggravates this problem. Asking health care providers to visit the family at home, on their own turf, is an effective strategy. Families are their own best advocates, and play a vital role in educating health care professionals about the impact that brain injury has on families. Everyone is so focused on the survivor that family issues are too often overlooked.

The Family as Expert

A family can be defined as a group of people who have a common history, and share responsibilities, and play many different roles in raising and educating children and meeting one another's needs. Since those outside the family do not share that history, they will often perceive a survivor's behaviour as winsome, or as rude and improper. They may have difficulty understanding why families regard appealing traits negatively, or why they tolerate behaviours that seem offensive. Example: A young man could be witty and entertaining; yet when he showed this behaviour in his mother's presence she frowned disapprovingly. When others pointed out her son's 'positive' traits, the mother suggested that they were being conned: 'He does that when he is unsure of himself, and if you fall for that you can't help him.'

Response to Survivors

It is helpful to model a way of communicating that praises the survivor's abilities and at the same time deals with the behaviour that is troublesome. This can be done in such a way as to demonstrate that the survivor is not emotionally fragile, and that families can be direct and open. It is usually not enough to scold or nag. It is far more effective to model the desired behaviour. 'This is the way *I* do it. Let me see *you* do it this way.' – and then ask the survivor to re-enact that behaviour in the family's presence. Also, it is important to ask directly what you want the survivor to do: 'I will pass you the peas again, and this time I want you to say thank you.' Survivors practise walking, holding a fork, dressing, and so on, yet practising social skills is often overlooked.

When the needs of the survivor clash with the needs of the family, the family must feel empowered to decide what has priority. Expecting survivors to make room for the needs of others encourages self-respect and allows them to experience being a 'real' family member, and not simply someone who must be babied or feared.

What Families Need to Know

Families profit from education about the medical aspects of brain injury, but this knowledge in itself is not enough. Knowing that damage to a certain brain structure results in poor judgment does not help you know what to do about it. In this case the family has to decide for the survivor. It is important to understand what factors in the environment lead to behavioural difficulties. Is the family expecting too much or too little? What can the survivor do successfully? What are the conditions that contribute to a good quality of life? Is there a balance between work, play, and social life? Who decides what role brain injury will have on family life? Should the survivor decide? Should the family decide? Should it be a mutual decision?

Though it is always advantageous for the survivor to participate in decisions when able, there are situations where the family must be in charge and make clear, firm decisions.

A Community of Families

Brain injury support groups are of immense benefit to families, and help them overcome feelings of being alone with their problems. Groups composed of families who 'have been there' provide a non-judgmental setting for exploring thoughts and feelings, as well as coping styles. This is as true during crisis management as it is when adjusting to chronic disability. Families are empowered when they realize that they can adjust their own coping efforts to fit changing circumstances. Support groups provide a base for understanding the emotional reactions that all families have when managing a crisis. Further, they help families decide what role they can play in their injured member's recovery, whether with health care providers or with the survivor directly. Knowing when to intervene and when to stand by, and how to negotiate, and when and how to elicit help, are important skills that can be learned.

Summary

Every family is a social system in which the whole is greater than the sum of its parts. What affects one part affects the whole, and what affects the whole affects each part. Families become organized in new ways in coping with a brain-injured member. With brain injury there are usually behavioural or cognitive difficulties that do not change or change very little. The family is at risk if its options are focused too narrowly on the survivor's needs and deficits or (at the other extreme) if it expects the survivor to 'sink or swim.' The emotional impact of brain injury changes the way family members relate to one another, sometimes in unexpected ways. All subsystems in the family are affected, and this results in major and minor role changes. The family has a vital role to play in educating itself, extended family members, health care providers, and others about the impact that brain injury has on spouses, parents, and siblings.

If the family is to resume its normal development, it must address the survivor's needs without neglecting its own. This requires planning for the future, which includes all members of the family; decision-making processes that are not hostage to illness-generated demands; relief from chronic anxiety and caretaking responsibilities; and the use of problem-solving approaches that fit changing circumstances.

13. Legal Issues Following Brain Injury

R. Brian Webster, BA, LLB

This is an introduction to legal issues, some or all of which will likely face survivors of traumatic brain injury or their families. I raise these issues and discuss them briefly with the expectation that readers will perhaps *note them* on first reading and then consider them again as the need arises. Discussion of these issues could fill a textbook by itself, so obviously this is just an introduction – something to make you aware when the issues require decisions or actions about which you must consult a lawyer. I can't overstate the importance of this principle. This is at most a guide. It is essential to contact a competent lawyer for advice.

I refer to the 'family' in this chapter because traumatic brain injury affects not just the survivor but the entire family. When considering legal issues (and possibly all issues), it is best that the survivor and family work together, each supporting the other. This will make understanding these issues and the burden of dealing with them far more bearable. I use 'his' when I refer to survivors of traumatic brain injury because most people who suffer traumatic brain injury (as opposed to other forms of brain injury) are male. For balance, I will use 'she' when referring to lawyers.

Do We Need a Lawyer?

There are few absolutes following traumatic brain injury, but one of them is that the survivor or his family *should*, and probably *will* eventually, consult a lawyer about some issue arising from the injury. Very soon after the injury, the family should consider whether some legal action may be required to *protect* the survivor or to *enhance* the quality of his life after recovery. Although you may not ultimately need a lawyer's services, a good lawyer will advise you whether the circumstances require ongoing legal assistance. Many lawyers do not charge for initial consultations.

If the traumatic brain injury was caused by the behaviour of another person, that person may be responsible in law to the survivor. Consult a lawyer with all possible speed to see that evidence is not lost, that the case is not prejudiced, and that no action is omitted that may compromise the survivor's options. The lawyer may state that there is no case, but at least the family will have that knowledge. There is no worse scenario than a lawyer having to tell a family there *might* have been a case but the witnesses have disappeared, or the evidence was destroyed because of time delay. Even if a lawyer is not needed immediately, contact has been made with one for later, if a need should arise.

Choosing the Right Lawyer

Choosing the right lawyer is fairly simple: hire a specialized lawyer, sometimes now called a *neuro-lawyer*. Do not hire a long-time family friend. Do get the names of three lawyers that your Brain Injury Association recommends, and interview all three in their offices. Ask these questions:

- How much of your practice involves traumatic brain injury?
- How long have you been doing cases involving traumatic brain injury?
- Have you attended or presented at any conferences on traumatic brain injury?
- May I have the name of one or two clients I could speak to?
- What is your basic philosophy or method of handling cases involving traumatic brain injury?

Choose the lawyer you feel most confident with after these meetings. Your Brain Injury Association has probably given you three good people to start with, so the answers to the questions themselves are not nearly as critical as how you *feel* about the lawyer.

If you lose confidence in a lawyer you have hired, there is no reason why you cannot change lawyers. The new lawyer will handle all the details involved with the changeover.

In most jurisdictions the issues arising from a traumatic brain injury are resolved through some form of litigation. *Litigation* is the system of resolving accident cases (or negligence cases) through court proceedings. Exceptions to this are *no-fault* systems and workers' compensation systems.

Survivors of brain injury and their families may be involved in litigation or in less controversial legal issues such as competency hearings, contracts, and estate planning. Sometimes disputes arise that do not directly involve proof of the injury, but that still involve an understanding of the injury and its consequences. Example: criminal cases. The same lawyer that you carefully chose at the beginning should be able to help with all these matters; if not, she can find someone else, and provide a briefing for you.

All neuro-lawyers will have acquired some technical knowledge about brain injury, but of course they are not physicians or psychologists. You have a right to expect that your lawyer has a working knowledge of the effects of traumatic brain injury, as well as a genuine interest in learning about your particular difficulty. A neuro-lawyer should be comfortable with you, and you with her. There should be an easy relationship where you are accepted and where you feel comfortable and respected by all. You should expect good communication (including copies of correspondence) and prompt personal access to the lawyer. You should expect her to give you her home number.

You should expect a neuro-lawyer to have a wide variety of experts available to assist. You should expect her to be an advocate for you, but a realistic one who does not make unrealistic promises. You should expect to pay legal fees based on a clear agreement with her. This may be based on a fee for time spent, or on a percentage of money actually recovered.

If you are making a claim to establish the injury and obtain damages, you should expect help now, but you should understand that settlement or money may not come for two to four years after the injury. You should expect the lawyer to be available to assist you in all aspects, including ensuring that you get very good independent advice concerning investments and your settlement.

The Nature of the Legal Process – Litigation

Most juridical systems, whether they involve courts or no-fault agencies, require the survivor or his representative to initiate a claim for either rehabilitation or compensation, and to follow that claim through, advocating each step as necessary. Some workers' compensation systems require matters be settled by a court; others forbid access to courts. All, however, require a filed claim followed by persistent advocacy.

All systems require the claim to be filed within some specified period of time. The process starts by filing the proper claim, and proceeds through various exchanges of information and documents up to the point of resolution. Failing satisfactory resolution, there may be an opportunity to appeal.

In cases involving civil litigation, each party must commence proceedings by issuing a writ or some similar document; then, as matters progress, they have an obligation to the other party to disclose relevant documents and information. These documents include medical records, school records, and tax returns. In most North American jurisdictions, each party in a civil case may conduct an oral cross-examination of the opposing party on relevant issues. These examinations, or depositions, are crucial as the questions and answers are admissible as evidence at the trial.

In cases involving survivors of traumatic brain injury, it is important to consider whether the survivor is able to answer questions reliably, or at all, under oath.

The litigation process proceeds over a period of months or years to the point of settlement – or failing that, to trial. A trial may be in front of a judge alone, or a judge and jury. At the time of trial, each party (plaintiff or defendant) has an opportunity to call witnesses before the court to testify regarding relevant matters. This may be evidence as to how someone has changed as a result of the injury or as to other functional losses. Witnesses are cross-examined by opposing counsel. The opposite party (the defence) then has an opportunity to lead its case, and its witnesses are likewise subject to cross-examination. Finally, arguments are addressed to the court concerning the evidence and the law, and then the court renders its judgment or the jury its verdict.

In cases involving serious traumatic brain injury, the court will expect expert opinions concerning the injury itself, the rehabilitation program, the need for continuing care or rehabilitation, lost income (both past and future), and any impairments of function. Final predictions of outcome, called prognoses, are submitted. The expert witnesses may testify and be cross-examined.

Typically, lay witnesses are persons who knew the survivor both before and after the injury, and who are capable of describing changes they have observed.

From the point at which the claim has been filed until its final resolution, the process usually includes a defence lawyer, whose duty is to reduce the amount of money paid. Sometimes the adversary is the adjuster in the insurance system or workers' compensation system, and that person's role may be a little difficult to discern immediately.

If at any stage the claim or litigation is resolved by agreement, such an agreement is referred to as a settlement.

Whether serious brain injury involves access to the courts, or the insurance system, or the workers' compensation system, the survivor will require advice and advocacy.

Timing Is Everything

A lawyer should be consulted as soon as possible, *immediately* after the injury. The purpose of this consultation is to obtain advice and, if appropriate, gather key evidence before it disappears or is destroyed. If key evidence is lost, the claim may be lost, regardless of the type of system.

Commencing a claim can be a highly complicated process. At the first meeting, the lawyer can establish to whom a claim may be made, as well as time lines for steps that may be necessary. There will be deadlines for filing documents or issuing proceedings; these vary widely in different jurisdictions and between various systems. You can be assured that with each potential claim, in each jurisdiction, there will be a deadline for filing *something*, and that failing to meet such deadlines may close the door to help forever. Find out these dates, and keep track of them.

Some jurisdictions provide protection for survivors of brain injury against the expiry of time limits because the survivor may not be legally competent following the injury, but relying on this is risky. It must not be assumed that because a survivor is helpless the law will protect him – that is not always the case.

Speed is essential for starting claims, but may be dangerous when it comes to settling them. Obviously, traumatic brain injuries take time to heal, and rehabilitation is also slow: It takes still more time to assess losses accurately and to predict future outcomes and needs. I suggest that an average of two to four years post-injury is necessary. Calculating future financial needs requires answering certain questions, including these:

- Will the survivor require continuing therapy, rehabilitation, and/ or care?
- If so, how much care or rehabilitation, for what period of time, and at what expense?
- Will the survivor be able to work, and if so, will he earn more or less over his lifetime relative to what he would have earned without the effects of injury?

Clearly, answering these questions will require considerable time and professional assessment. No settlement should be made or trial take place unless the answers are available.

Remedies – An Introduction to Damages

It is a basic principle of Anglo-American law that someone who is injured due to the negligence of another is entitled to financial compensation to restore the injured person as fully as possible to the state he would have been in had the negligence not occurred. For negligence, read *fault* – the failure to be reasonably careful that you do not cause injury to someone else by your behaviour.

In a conventional legal system, when a person is injured by a person at fault, the wrongdoer may be found liable by a court to pay damages. The damages will usually be covered by the wrongdoer's insurance up to the value of the insurance policy limits.

Damages are considered under various categories. The two main groups are 'economic losses' and 'non-economic losses.' Non-economic losses relate to damages for pain and suffering, loss of function, and loss of enjoyment of life. In 1978 the Supreme Court of Canada set an artificial limit, thereafter to be adjusted by cost-of-living increases (see *Andrews V. Grand & Toy Alberta Ltd.*, [1978] 2 S.C.R. 229). The current limit is now about $250,000 (1996 dollars) for the most seriously injured person's non-economic losses. Awards for less serious injuries will be correspondingly smaller. In the United States there is no such ceiling. Even so, average awards for damages are very similar between England, Canada, and the United States.

The other main category of damages, 'economic losses,' relates to provable past and future financial losses. Typically damages include the following:

• Special damages – out-of-pocket expenses for which you have receipts.
• Past wage loss.
• Future loss of earnings – the present value of the loss of one's ability to earn income over a lifetime, whether in whole or in part.
• Past and future care – the present value of the expense of all rehabilitation and care that is reasonably necessary over a lifetime.
• Any other losses suffered by the injured person that are directly caused by the incident, including (in Canada) income taxes paid on interest earned on the funds invested for future care.

These categories understate the complexity of the proof required to support the damages. Establishing such proof often occupies an experienced lawyer for many weeks or months. The lawyer usually retains various experts to assist in preparing and presenting evidence to support the claim.

Damages are calculated at the time of settlement or trial, and are usually paid as a lump sum. This is a once-and-for-all figure. In the litigation process, any damage that is missed or unforeseen will never be recovered.

In a few systems, subsequent care needs may be considered, such as with an active workers' compensation file.

Some insurance companies advocate a change from lump sum to periodic payments so that those payments would cease if the recipient gets better (or dies). However, similar consideration is never suggested to *increase* payments if the need for care increases over time.

A lump sum settlement (but not a court-ordered judgment), may be partly 'structured.' The meaning of this will be described in the section on settlements.

The survivor and family will want to double-check to ensure the completeness of the budget for future care funds. Some suggestions for this follow:

- Keep a record of all expenditures since the accident.
- Arrive at a reasonable estimate of the amount of family time spent to care for the survivor.
- Make sure there is a co-ordinated, co-operative, and communicative rehabilitation team.
- Make sure there is a clear rehabilitation path before settlement, as well as a plan for after the settlement.
- Make sure the rehabilitation team and plan are managed by a competent case manager.
- Make sure the needs for different types of rehabilitation and care are realistically assessed now and into the future – changes will need to be made over time.
- Make sure earnings losses are carefully examined, and that documents are obtained and properly valued.

Doing all of the above will contribute to proper rehabilitation and reasonable prospects for ample rehabilitation and care after settlement. It is my experience that a co-operative and communicative team and case manager will improve rehabilitation and facilitate adequate damage assessment.

What Will This Cost ... How Do I Pay?

There are expenses involved in making a claim for damages. Legal costs will include everything reasonably necessary to bring the case to trial. The most obvious is the legal fee itself. These fees may be pay-as-you-go, or may be paid as a percentage when and *if* the case succeeds. This latter type is called a *contingent fee*. The contingent fee is the friend of the seriously injured and economically disadvantaged, because without this type of fee only insurance companies and the rich would be able to litigate serious cases. Contingent fees are outlawed in Ontario; even so, other 'arrangements' can be made to obtain a lawyer's help. Please ask. In the past, contingency fees were also prohibited in England. However, over the last two years, a 'Conditional Fee' has evolved that is based not on the damages recovered, but rather on the amount of costs recovered from a defendant's insurance company.

Other typical expenses include those necessary to collect evidence and investigate the facts, and to obtain the opinions of expert witnesses. (There are also myriad miscellaneous expenses.) Unless otherwise agreed, these expenses may be borne by the survivor or family regardless of the outcome of the case. Lawyers refer to these expenses as disbursements.

A case manager or rehabilitation co-ordinator may be necessary as well. This expense is necessary, in my view, to ensure the proper care of the survivor, to reduce the pressures on the family, and to ensure a cohesive and co-operative team approach to rehabilitation and care. If the insurer does not fund an *independent* professional rehabilitation manager, then the lawyer or family should. This usually will not be an employee of the insurance company.

Some of these litigation expenses may be recovered as *costs* following a successful trial or upon settlement. The amount recovered will vary. Some lawyers will accept part of the recovered costs as reimbursement for part of their fee. (Contingent fee agreements are of course negotiable, so I suggest you do just that – negotiate).

These costs vary tremendously between jurisdictions, but generally are between 10 and 40 per cent of legal fees plus disbursements.

Fault / No Fault

Earlier, I described the traditional legal process as one founded on the presence of negligence – that is, the person at fault should pay damages to the person he or she injured. There are disadvantages to a pure fault system, in that it may be some time before trial, with no interim financial assistance available. It is also possible that a person who injures himself will never receive compensation. Various jurisdictions have softened the edges of the fault system by offering immediate rehabilitation assistance. Still others have eliminated the concept of fault and pay reduced benefits to anyone who has been injured, regardless of fault. The most familiar no-fault systems are the various workers' compensation schemes. Each such scheme varies, and some still require litigation to settle the amount. Several American states tried a no-fault system for their general automobile insurance and have subsequently retreated, as has the province of Ontario. No-fault schemes are generally found too expensive, and are opposed by many disability advocacy groups.

In many jurisdictions there is a continuing debate about the wisdom of no-fault. Some people with straightforward and visible injuries may receive benefits more quickly through a no-fault system. However, survivors of traumatic brain injury and their families are in general agreement that they do not do well in a no-fault system, as these systems are usually designed to eliminate advocates, so that traumatic brain injury survivors are on their own.

A common characteristic of no-fault systems is that they provide immediate rehabilitation funding, to be dispensed by approved persons according to schedules and regulations. They also provide listed financial benefits, also administered by the same no-fault entity. There may or may not be any right of appeal, yet at the same time, access to the courts is usually stopped.

Another common characteristic of no-fault systems is there are no 'lump sum' payments. This means there is a continuing administration of, and therefore involvement with, the survivor's care. Immigrants from some countries with a less benevolent history of bureaucracy than our own find this an intrusion. Some families prefer to 'opt out' and take their loved one home and do the best they can without interference. Others cope well with a long-term dependence on bureaucracy.

In a *fault* system, most people carry insurance. Insurance, of course, is a contract whereby the person at fault is 'indemnified' (his losses are paid for him) by an insurance company, to which he has paid a premium. When an injured person sues the wrongdoer, that wrongdoer has insurance to pay for the claim. In most countries there are private insurance companies, but increasingly there are public schemes that offer basic coverage or that have replaced private insurers.

Also, some jurisdictions now provide compensation for criminal injuries, administered either through a workers' compensation authority or through some other independent body.

Limitation Dates

In every jurisdiction there is a date beyond which, depending on the legal issue, no claim may be made. This date is usually quite final. Do not let it go by because of inattention to business. Do not let it go by because you are preoccupied with issues of rehabilitation and care. The best approach is to retain counsel and have her watch the dates for you. These dates can be quite short for certain types of claims, so it is vital to get advice soon.

In principle, no one who is incapable of looking after his own affairs following a traumatic brain injury should be barred from a claim because of the expiry of a limitation date. If you have let the limitation slip by, do still consult a lawyer, because it may be possible to apply for an extension. This is by no means certain, however.

Jurisdictional Issues

When lawyers speak of 'jurisdiction,' they may be referring to the state, country, or province whose laws govern the apportionment of fault or the award of compensation. In Canada it is the law of the place where the incident occurred that governs the wrongdoing. Thus, if you are involved in an accident in British Columbia, it is the law of British Columbia that governs whether someone is at fault.

Typically, then, when someone is injured who is visiting from another place, matters need to be settled in the jurisdiction or location where the injury occurred. The best plan is to retain an expert near your home and have that person find the best expert in the distant jurisdiction. Be aware that there are very limited funds available in some places for any kind of medical or rehabilitation assistance. Many places offer a chequerboard of rehabilitation schemes. Some places are much better than others, so it is worth inquiring, as 'home' may not be the best place for rehabilitation or rehabilitation funding. Check this out.

The Team

The legal approach following brain injury should be a team approach. The neuro-lawyer is best thought of as the leader of a client-centred team that includes a case manager. *Legal* members of the team will include some, or all, of the following:

- The lawyer, perhaps with junior lawyers and legal assistants.
- Expert witnesses and economists (to prove lifetime values of economic losses).
- Actuary (to prove present value of future losses).
- Engineer (to reconstruct causes of vehicular or other accidents).
- Private investigator (to locate witnesses).

The *non-legal* members of the team may include neuropsychologists, speech and language pathologists, occupational therapists, physiotherapists, and physicians. The latter might include the family doctor, a neurosurgeon, a neurologist, a psychiatrist, and/or a physiatrist. Chapter 4 describes the roles these team members play.

This cohesive and co-operative team of qualified specialists not only will improve the outcome, but may well also reduce the burden on the survivor and his family. A good case manager whose primary focus is at all times on the survivor's rehabilitation, care, and recovery, is fundamental – not just as part of the rehabilitation process, but as part of the legal process.

Accessing Rehabilitation Funding

In Canada, the United Kingdom, and the United States, there is good medical care following traumatic brain injury. There is usually immediate institutional rehabilitation – for example, speech therapy and physiotherapy. But once the acute stage has passed, there is little public funding anywhere specifically for survivors of traumatic brain injury. Some services are available but these vary widely between countries and between urban and rural locations, and are often very expensive. Professionals offering services for general neurological rehabilitation may have to be located and accessed. In some instances they may be available only for a fee. Rehabilitation must of course continue well beyond the acute stage. If the case manager can find the services, someone will need to fund them.

Generally, these services can only be obtained through private funds or insurance funds. In my experience the best way of accessing these services, and the funds to pay, is through a family-instructed rehabilitation case manager. This person is usually expert at accessing the funding and finding the services. Brain injury associations and hospital social workers may also assist. All of these people have developed expertise at finding paths through the government, health care, insurance, and litigation bureaucracies. It is not impossible for the family to do the same, but it is burdensome, and better done by others.

Subrogation

Private insurers, and sometimes public agencies and employers, may require that money they have paid as benefits to the survivor (such as disability benefits) be recovered back from the 'guilty party.' This concept is referred to as the *right of subrogation*. This is important, because sometimes people forget that interim disability payments will have to be returned to the insurance company from the final settlement. Sometimes survivors forget to do this, and are themselves sued by the insurance company. It is important to be aware of what you are signing when you seek interim benefits. It is best to seek advice so that you do not promise to return money you do not have. Discuss this with your lawyer.

Competency – The Concept of Guardianship

We all understand that young children are presumed incapable of bargaining away their rights, or of maintaining and settling lawsuits or entering into serious adult contracts. It is also understandable that children cannot finalize settlements or instruct lawyers. The same concept may apply to persons who have lost the ability to manage their own affairs due to a serious brain injury. We refer to children as 'infants,' and we refer to those who cannot manage their own affairs as 'incompetent.' The problem is, as we all know, that children vary tremendously as to their competence, as do people who have had a brain injury. Once children reach the age of majority they are presumed completely capable and able to manage their own affairs. It is assumed that an adult's capability continues even after a severe brain injury unless someone has applied to a court, usually upon the sworn evidence of two doctors, for a declaration that the person is incapable of managing his or her own affairs.

Upon such a declaration being made, a person, typically a family member (or failing that, a public official), is appointed to act as the *committee* of the person suffering the disability. A committee is a form of agent. One of the things a committee may do is act as a guardian for the purposes of litigation.

Unfortunately, in most jurisdictions the issue of competence is still perceived in black-and-white terms: a person is either competent or incompetent. However, it is now becoming recognized that there is a middle ground where persons *may* be competent given sufficient help and support. Various jurisdictions are now contemplating complex adult guardianship rules to try to cover this middle ground.

Until those rules are enacted and operating in your jurisdiction, the best way to avoid problems is to act together as a family; this will allow you to provide strength, safety, and support not only to the survivor but to one another, without necessarily removing all the rights of the person with diminished abilities. Unfortunately, this is only possible if the survivor is at least partially competent.

It is a very difficult decision for a family to ask for a declaration of incompetency. It may be seen as giving up. I suggest that it is often the correct step and one that should be made promptly. Some people may see it as the removal of the survivor's basic civil rights, but it also should be seen as a means to protect the survivor against many dangers. It is best if the committee or guardian is someone in the family whose commitment to the injured person is long-term and unconditional.

The question of guardianship must be canvassed at the time a lawsuit is commenced. It must be considered again when an issue arises as to whether the survivor can give oral evidence; and finally, it must be revisited at the time of settlement.

Settlement

We often use the term 'settlement' loosely. Settlement really refers to entering into an agreement – that is, a deal by which a case is settled, often involving a payment of money. It is consensual.

'Judgment,' on the other hand, is an award of damages by a judge or jury. It is not arrived at by agreement, and in most jurisdictions it is paid once and for all, in the form of a lump sum.

Settlement provides some opportunities to plan for the future, as one may be able to negotiate a *structured settlement*. A structured settlement is an arrangement whereby an agreed payment of money is used to purchase an annuity from another insurance company. That insurance company then promises to pay a blended payment of principal and interest to the survivor on a monthly basis and on terms that are agreed. A structured settlement can be a valuable component of any planned settlement process. The question of whether to take a structured settlement rather than lump sum, and on what terms, is highly complex and requires professional advice from an actuary, as well as legal counsel. These complex settlements are permanent and cannot be changed. Remember that in times of economic and social change, the settlement does not change; and that in times of changing personal needs, no amendment is possible.

Yet at the same time, such inflexibility is the *strength* of the structured settlement. It cannot be stolen (other than by one payment at a time), nor can it be wasted on a bad investment. It may not be pledged at a bank to secure a loan. It comes routinely and on the terms arranged.

Another component of a planned settlement should be a competent financial planner. Choosing a good one may be crucial. I suggest someone who has experience, who is independent and professional, and whose job is managing funds, not brokering. All of this suggests that well-meaning friends are often not the best qualified to give financial advice, nor are familiar figures like bankers. It may be better to pay a fee and hire a manager, instead of paying a commission and hiring a broker.

The lawyer and the family should double-check every element of this final process. The case manager, having prepared a cost of future care, should prepare a budget that reflects the amount available and the monthly needs for care, rehabilitation, housing, and so on. A structured settlement may well be an important part of that budget.

It is important not to forget income tax issues in this planning process. Funds that are owned by a survivor and that receive interest income will bear income tax. Structured settlement payments will not. If this is not considered, there may be unpleasant surprises at tax time.

There will be investment issues to consider during the settlement. Example: Is it appropriate to buy a house? Also, ways must be found to protect the survivor from being taken advantage of. At the same time, the funds are intended to provide proper care for the survivor – to enhance the quality of his life – and should not be hoarded. Again, a case manager may be invaluable to when it comes to ensuring that payments are actually used for care.

Marriage Agreements and Estate Planning

Marriage agreements should be considered to protect the settlement. Marriages are at risk following traumatic brain injury, and arrangements should be made to ensure that the settlement will stay with the survivor. As well, there are issues of estate planning to consider. The parents and grandparents of the survivor will wish to consider establishing a trust, or some other arrangement by which they may pass on their estate to the survivor. The survivor may wish to make plans so that he can pass on funds to his children. All of this requires specialized planning, which in turn requires competent legal counsel.

Children: Some Special Problems

When the injury is to a child, there arise a number of special legal and other issues. It is even more difficult to predict outcomes when the survivor is a child. In particular, it is hard to predict exactly how a loss suffered by a child may manifest itself in economic terms. It is therefore crucial to address extensively the rehabilitation needs of the child; it is equally crucial to wait until the results come clear. It may be a number of years before anyone has a clear idea of the outcome. For example, until the child has finished high school it may be impossible to say whether he will be able to find competitive employment.

Insurance companies greatly prefer to pay out a child's claim as soon as possible, because this minimizes their risk. It is difficult to decide whether to accept a settlement that must go into trust. Does one wait until the case becomes clearer?

Sometimes parents were involved in the child's injury. Parents should be aware that the insurance company may add them as defendants. This is done for tactical reasons, but also in some cases because the parents may bear some degree of fault. In many jurisdictions, if more than one person is at fault, each person is jointly responsible for all of the loss. Thus, an insurance company may be able to bring in another insurance company to share the expense. For that reason, when considering who will act as the litigation guardian for a child, consider a near relative rather than a parent.

Miscellaneous Issues

LOSS OF PRIVACY

There is an almost complete loss of privacy rights for a plaintiff's medical, vocational, and other relevant documents and records. It is assumed that when a person makes a claim for a serious personal injury, he has voluntarily waived confidentiality. This may even apply to conversations between doctor and patient, but it certainly applies to doctors' records. One should anticipate this.

CRIMINAL

The criminal justice system is not particularly forgiving of those who suffer behavioural problems following traumatic brain injury. If they are not insane and are found fit to stand trial, survivors of brain injuries will be dealt with like any other person before the court. It is best to make a serious effort to keep persons with brain injury problems out of the criminal court system. If a survivor does get embroiled, experts used in the civil justice system are useful in criminal proceedings.

14. Leisure and Recreation

Anne Sulzberger, Dip. RT
Charles Killingsworth, PhD

What Is Leisure? What Role Does It Play?

Leisure plays a vital regenerative role in our lives. By participating in leisure or recreation, we express our individuality – social, physical, emotional, spiritual, and intellectual. The activities we pursue reflect our personal values and beliefs; for example, an individual who enjoys being physically active will express this through activities such as sports, walking, and exercise. These pursuits may or may not involve others, depending on the personality and needs of the individual. Awareness and experience of leisure directly affects quality of life. Few of us find fulfillment solely from our work. More typically, work is what allows us to pursue activities that give meaning and joy to our lives. These activities generally involve opportunities to share our lives with people whom we value.

It is through our recreation and leisure interests that we make friends, keep physically and mentally healthy, relieve stress, and find peace and tranquility. For many of us, the interests and activities we pursue constitute our 'raison d'etre.'

The Effect of a Brain Injury on Leisure Participation

The effects of a brain injury can be subtle or pronounced. In either case, learning to adapt and compensate is a challenge for the survivor and his or her caregivers. Survivors are too often forced into 'retirement' at an age when their friends are working, going to school, getting married, and generally leading 'normal' lives. People with brain injury may no longer be able to participate in their old leisure interests due to physical, cognitive, and psychosocial changes. They will need to adjust to a different level of ability.

Cognitive changes – to memory, learning, orientation, judgment, information processing, initiative, and motivation – affect the survivor's ability to participate in recreation. Factors affecting participation include these: an inability to remember plans, people, names, and places; an inability to come up with and follow through on ideas; the need for support due to limited attention span; and an inability to get around without getting lost. Impaired judgment and reasoning can put individuals at risk, especially in unfamiliar settings and with unfamiliar people. The support needed to soften the impact of these changes can be extensive and often must be provided by the family or other caregivers.

Physical changes such as decreased endurance, visual deficits (double-vision, restricted vision, inability to track, loss of vision to one side), reduced physical abilities, and (for some) reliance on a wheelchair or communication aids mean the individual will need to adapt in a variety of ways. This will often involve: learning to pace activities; seeking out accessible facilities, transportation, and activities; and letting go of old interests and learning new ones that are more suitable.

Psychosocial changes are often the most devastating. Inappropriate social behaviours often make it difficult for the survivor to be accepted, and result in old friends withdrawing from the person's life. As a result, the person's family or caregivers become the primary source of socialization; this often leads to social isolation. This isolation can lead to yet more cognitive and emotional problems and, for some, depression. People are social beings by nature, and need to have others with whom they can share their experiences. Everyone needs social interaction. People whose behaviour is 'disinhibited' tend to drive others away, and some programs are unwilling to accept them as members. These issues must be managed if we are to ensure the survivor's long-term adjustment.

Following are some suggestions for improving socialization and a personal sense of self-worth and self-esteem (this list is not exhaustive):

- Increase the survivor's opportunities to interact with others – especially those with whom he or she would want to socialize. (Later in the chapter, we will discuss how to identify interests and resources.) In the process of locating people and activities of interest to the survivor, we may find others who will be willing to support him or her in various activities. This will broaden the scope of experiences for the person to enjoy; it will also increase the survivor's exposure to persons with similar interests. For the caregiver, this can mean a much-needed break.
- Call your local Brain Injury Association for advice, information, and assistance. They should be able to tell you about recreation programs and services, and suggest professionals who can provide guidance and teach skills.
- Rebuilding a positive sense of self, and a social network, is a lengthy and difficult process. People with brain injury must often begin at square one to relearn an old activity. They will need instruction and constant practice in order to rebuild confidence and skill. They will have to repeat the process again and again with each new challenge, and this involves caregivers providing time and support. Some attempts will result in success, some in failure. However, both are part of learning; the hardest part will be to get back up and try again.

  Survivors may also have to relearn social skills. Repeated opportunities to socialize will enhance this process. It is important to remember, however, that every survivor relearns social skills at a different pace. For some, just daily care needs will be all they can handle, while for others, social clubs, libraries, sports clubs, and so on will be appropriate. Reinforcing appropriate social behaviour is very important. Often, subtle cues can be used to remind the person to slow down or back off – for example, a tug on the ear to let them know they are talking too fast. The cues will often be graduated; that is, they will be obvious at first and gradually become less so. The repetition and reinforcement can sometimes be frustrating and aggravating. Working out the parameters with survivors is beneficial. They will feel that they have some control over the choice of cues, and they will also feel some responsibility for them. Following up after positive and negative experiences helps. For many, this follow-up will need to be immediately after, so that they can remember the details of the situation.

- Break tasks into small, simple steps (it is amazing how many steps are required to drink a glass of water). Each step achieved will provide a sense of accomplishment as well as an incentive to move forward. We all need to feel good about what we do and how well we do. When we feel successful, we gain self-confidence and begin the process of rebuilding our self-esteem. Remember also that the survivor should feel good about reaching his or her own personal best – and you should feel good along with them. It is sometimes difficult to accept that a loved one is unable to meet our expectations. Let the survivor be your guide. We also sometimes need to allow them to struggle. It may seem 'cruel' to watch someone struggle with a task; however, this is part of learning, and we must be prepared to step back and let this process occur.

- Establish roles for the survivor to fill. Everyone has roles: father, son, friend, worker, volunteer, and so on. We place a great deal of value on the roles we have, and we perceive those roles as a measure of our self-worth. Many of us associate our self-worth with the work we do, but many brain-injured individuals will be unable to return to 'work.' A volunteer role may help fill this gap and at the same time provide opportunities for the survivor to be with others and contribute to a meaningful cause. Volunteering may also make it easier for the survivor to return to work farther down the road.

What Happens to the Caregiver and Family?

The demands of caregiving take their toll on all aspects of the caregiver's life, especially in the area of recreation and leisure, because of the amount of time, energy, and resources needed to care for the person with the brain injury. Because in most families leisure receives less attention than work, it is sometimes considered less important in helping family members cope with their situation. There seems to be less time available to take the children to their various after-school involvements (sports, music, dance, and so on), and less time for the caregiver to be involved in his or her own leisure activities. But again, things can be done to encourage continued involvement in recreational interests. This may, however, involve setting priorities and being more selective in those involvements. The only certainty is that each individual member of the family, including the person with the brain injury, needs recreation time.

Developing a Meaningful Leisure Lifestyle

Developing a meaningful leisure lifestyle is a challenge. The first step in meeting it is to develop an understanding of the person and his or her values. It is also important to remember that for the survivor, as for everyone, this is a life-long process. Everyone should try to maintain an open mind and experiment with new and different activities.

What interests did the survivor have pre-injury? When, where, and with whom did the survivor participate in these interests? What kind of people did the person like to associate with? What did he or she get out of participating in their interests? Why did these activities give the person enjoyment? What makes this person tick? What is his or her current financial situation? Answering these questions builds a profile of what the person is *about*. If the person had a keen interest in classical music before the injury, it is highly unlikely that he or she will suddenly be interested in Country & Western. You need also to consider the interests you *shared* with the individual. If you have been through rehabilitation, you already have encountered a recreation therapist who assisted in developing this foundation. If you are having problems and need help, don't hesitate to call that person now. Most often he or she will be more than willing to offer advice and guidance. A brief Leisure Needs Profile is provided in Figure 14.1 at the end of this chapter. It should help you discover the leisure interests and needs of the individual with the brain injury; it may also help you understand your own leisure lifestyle.

Once you have a basic understanding of the survivor's interests, the process begins of identifying those which can be adapted, relearned, and supported. In some cases the individual will not want to participate in previous interests. This should be respected; however, an activity similar in nature may be appropriate. Perhaps an adapted form of the previous activity – for example, wheelchair sports – would be appropriate.

Learning what the individual has for resources at home and in the community is very important. Finances certainly play a role and need to be reviewed. There are many free or low-cost activities one can pursue, such as walks on the beach, going to the library, playing cards or games, and joining a community organization such as a stamp club. Your local recreation department may be willing to reduce its fees for individuals with disabilities or who have a limited income. Also, many recreation departments have a special needs worker on staff who will be able to help identify suitable activities and find additional supports where required. Many theatres, restaurants, and so on offer reduced cost evenings such as $3.00 Tuesdays and two-for-one meals. Don't be afraid to ask about these allowances and special offers – the worst you will hear is 'no.' If you live in a community that sells 'entertainment' books or similar, you may want to consider buying these.

It is very helpful to develop a *resource book* to keep track of leisure information. It not only keeps the information available for future reference, but also acts as a compensatory tool for individuals with cognitive problems, such as memory loss.

The resource book should include information on the following: personal interests, equipment and supplies needed, costs, locations, days and times (including total time needed), contact people, seasonal information, transportation requirements, accessibility, and support requirements. The resource book can be whatever format works best: a computer program, recipe cards, or a binder.

Keeping a *diary* of daily activities can be very helpful. Our memories form the individuals we are. An inability to remember what we did the day before, or even an hour earlier, can be very frustrating; it also limits our self-awareness and awareness of the world. It is through our life experiences that we learn, and define our lives.

Volunteer support can help relieve some of the stress on the care-giver; it can also broaden the survivor's social network. Volunteer agencies do not usually assign volunteers to individuals; this needs to be pursued through local recreation departments, clubs, or service organizations or agencies. Volunteers may also be found in your net-work of friends and colleagues. It is important for caregivers to remember that if the injury had not occurred, the survivor would have friends in the same age group and be involved in interests suit-able to their personality, age, and ability. The burden of care is a heavy one, and caregivers must find ways to safeguard their own well-being as well as the survivor's. Whenever possible, involve-ments in social networks and activities consistent with the person's age, personality, and interests should be encouraged.

Accessibility, in all meanings of the word, is very important. Building codes now have provisions for accessible entrances, wash-rooms, and seating. Even so, it is important to check this out before going on outings. An in-person visit is sometimes the most time- and cost-saving approach. Accessible transportation is now available in most cities and towns. Individuals who are not in wheelchairs can also utilize these services if they are required for safety or other rea-sons. Contact your local transit office, recreation department, or Brain Injury Association for assistance in locating these services.

Attitude is a far greater challenge. Peoples' awareness and accep-tance of individuals with disabilities has greatly increased. Educa-tion and interaction together change attitudes. Don't be afraid to advocate on behalf of yourself or the person you are with.

Long-term Benefits of Leisure Activities for Persons with Brain Injury

While the concept of including people with disabilities in commu-nity recreation and leisure activities is not a new one, it is only recently that this has become a major focus for individuals with more severe disabilities, including brain injury. The Americans with Disabilities Act (1991) in the United States, 'the Universal Dec-laration of Human Rights proclaimed by the United Nations, the 'Closer to Home' initiative of the government of British Columbia, the de-institutionalization of persons with disabilities in Canada and the United States, the move to a managed care approach to health care in the United States, and similar initiatives have forced the issue, both within communities and with service providers. As a result, a variety of resources have been created to help meet the needs of people with disabilities and bring them into community services.

Problems have been encountered in integrating people with disabilities with other citizens in community programs and services. Besides the architectural barriers encountered in many community facilities, there are attitudinal barriers that create perhaps even larger problems. Both of these problems are being dealt with, and as a result both non-disabled people and those with disabilities are reaping the benefits. Better facilities, greater options, and increased tolerance of differences have come of the movement to include *all* people in recreation and leisure services.

Following are some of the benefits of recreation for people with brain injury: a greater acceptance of the survivor into the community; improved self-esteem and self-acceptance; a greater sense of self-worth; and the saving of taxpayers' dollars through decreased duplication of services. Recreation enables people to escape their daily routines; it facilitates relaxation, teaches new skills and reteaches lost ones, and improves cognitive functioning. All of these things contribute to a healthier and happier lifestyle for both the survivor and the caregivers.

Recreation is vital to fostering socialization and developing friendships, so it is very important for the brain-injured survivor and the caregivers to keep up their involvement in such activities. This involvement should follow two main avenues: identifying activities that can be done as a family; and identification of activities that each family member can do *away* from other family members – that is, with peers or friends, or alone. Working and playing together as a family is very important, but it is just as important for each of us to have 'personal time,' and time away from our family roles. The *Leisure Self-Evaluation* (Figure 14.1), provides a brief tool to help you look at yours or your family members' leisure and begin the process of developing a meaningful leisure lifestyle.

FIGURE 14.1 **Leisure Self-Evaluation***

What do I want from leisure experiences?

_____ to do something meaningful
_____ to contribute to my community
_____ to continue learning
_____ to be creative/expressive
_____ to relax
_____ to be able to do what I want
_____ a sense of accomplishment
_____ to challenge myself

_____ to spend time with
     friends/family
_____ to by physically active
_____ to use/learn new skills
_____ to make friends
_____ to laugh & have fun
_____ to feel needed / wanted

Leisure Interests (indicate if you have done, are presently doing, want to do)

Social

_____ Visiting/talking to friends
_____ Joining a club/group
_____ Making social phone calls
_____ Eating out
_____ Church groups
_____ Going to movies

Creative

_____ Crafts
_____ Painting/drawing
_____ Cooking/Baking
_____ Fly Tying
_____ Writing stories/music
_____ Wine/Beer Making

Physical

_____ Playing sports
_____ Going for walks
_____ Swimming
_____ Gardening
_____ Fishing

Intellectual

_____ Reading the newspaper
_____ Going to the library
_____ Discussing different topics
_____ Taking a course
_____ Reading

What other activities am I interested in? (Think about outdoor & indoor, seasonal activities, things done alone/at home, things done with others) _

_____
_____
_____
_____
_____
_____
_____

What makes it difficult for me to do the things I am interested in?

____ Don't feel like doing anything	____ Too busy
____ Work/school is a priority	____ No transportation
____ Not enough money	____ Lack the skills needed
____ No one to go with	____ Don't know where to start
____ I can't get started	____ Social situations are awkward

Other _____

_____

*Adapted from *Leisure Your Lifestyle*, Ontario Ministry of Tourism and Recreation (1980), and Richard Shack's *Recreation Is Where You Find It*.

Where to Find Resources

The extent and variety of resources available will depend on a number of factors, including the size of community, the number of caregivers and persons with a brain injury in the local area, and sources of funding. Smaller communities are sometimes more supportive, as they feel a sense of responsibility to their community members.

At the local level, the resources may include:

- Support groups
- Religious organizations
- Recreation and parks departments
- Schools
- Corporations
- Advocacy organizations
- Service groups
- Social services departments
- Clubs

At the state/provincial level, resources may include:

- Departments of Parks and Recreation
- Rehabilitation/social services
- Advocacy organizations
- Colleges/universities
- Brain Injury Associations
- Stroke Foundation
- Corporations
- Therapeutic recreation services
- Adapted sports groups

At the federal level, resources may include:

- Advocacy organizations
- Therapeutic recreation associations
- Health/welfare departments
- Recreation and parks associations
- Recreation and parks departments

How does one get started? Decide what you want to do. Then start asking questions: Why do you want to do it? Where can you get information? Where is the activity done? When is the activity done? What does it cost? What do I need in order to do the activity? How will I get to the activity? Do I need support to participate?

Now, set a date on which you would like to begin, and search out the information you need. If you need help, ask friends, call your recreation department, or ask your local support group.

15. The Family as Caregiver

Sonia Acorn, RN, PhD

No longer are health professionals the only providers of care. Today, with an increase in the number of people with disabilities and chronic illnesses, and the growing number of elderly, many people find themselves in the role of 'caregiver.' This is evident in the vital role that family caregivers play in providing care to survivors of brain injury. However, those who provide care to a family member should be aware of the long-term effects that caregiving has on their own health. It is important for them to take steps to safeguard their own physical and emotional well-being, while providing much-needed support to the family member. The continuing stress associated with caring for a brain-injured survivor over an extended period of time can lead to burnout on the part of the caregiver. Another common result of caregiving is social isolation. In this chapter, we will discuss stress, burnout, and social isolation, as well as the valuable role that support groups can play in helping the caregiver cope with the responsibility of caregiving.

Caregivers

Most caregiving roles fall to women. In a survey of family caregivers of brain-injured survivors in British Columbia, 95 per cent of the caregivers were women, about half of these were in their forties. Within the family unit, it is women who have traditionally provided care to children and to family members who are ill. Many women assume these caregiving responsibilities on top of an already busy lifestyle, thus placing themselves in danger of stress and burnout. Because most caregivers are women, we will use 'she' in this chapter when referring to them. For the sake of balance, survivors will be referred to as 'he.'

Caregiving is a major responsibility that can involve anything from doing someone else's shopping, to helping perform the various activities of daily living. The caregiving role can be both stressful and burdensome, and caregivers usually experience a wide range of emotions. Feelings of conflict are common because the role of the caregiver often represents a change in a relationship that was previously more reciprocal (example: the transformation from the mother of an *independent* adult son to the mother of a *dependent* adult son). The caregiver may become socially isolated as she devotes a proportion of her time to caring for the survivor. Also, caregivers may feel guilt, anger, and/or resentment over the situation in which they find themselves, and may become fatigued in the caregiving role. These factors, while understandable, can contribute to caregiver stress and (eventually) burnout. Steps need to be taken to alleviate these feelings and thereby ensure the overall well-being of the caregiver.

Stress, Burnout, and Isolation

Stress is the felt response to pressures and tensions in the environment. *Burnout*, which can result from prolonged periods of stress, is a feeling of being completely overwhelmed and unrewarded, and can contribute to depression and physical illness in the caregiver. A person who is caring for a brain-injured survivor, and is not receiving needed assistance, and has no opportunity to share experiences with others, is in danger of suffering burnout. Feeling completely exhausted at the end of the day, with no emotional or physical strength remaining to care for oneself, is a sign of burnout. This is a warning signal to the caregiver that she needs to be concerned about her own physical and emotional needs and take corrective measures to ensure her continued health. It is important for caregivers to recognize situations that may lead to burnout and develop suitable methods of coping.

Stresses experienced by the family caregiver may include the following:

- Physical strain associated with providing care.
- Isolation and loneliness.
- Lack of sleep.
- Emotional strain associated with the physical and behavioural changes that have occurred in the loved one.

Personal strategies to cope with stress include these:

- Arrange quiet time – reading, walking, relaxation exercises, or gardening.
- Talk with someone – often just verbalizing feelings or letting off steam to a good listener can help.
- Get more information – know as much as you can about the brain injury and the resources that are available to you.
- Ask for help from relatives; caregiving is a hard job to do alone.
- Use home care nurses or respite care, if available.
- Talk with others who are caregivers. They can offer you tips and techniques for coping.

Sometimes the methods an individual uses to cope with stress are ineffective. For example, a woman who is feeling pressured may go on a shopping spree, eat or drink too much, or lash out at someone. These reactions do little to control the stress, and often end up compounding an already stressful situation. *Take time to care for yourself; it is essential to your well-being!*

There is a real danger of caregivers becoming *socially isolated*. This isolation usually arises because the caregiver can't leave the home, because the survivor cannot be left unattended. Also, there is a general tendency to gradually withdraw from social activities, due to the time commitment required to care for the survivor and the physical and emotional exhaustion resulting from the caregiving responsibilities. Many caregivers feel they are alone – that no one understands or cares about their situation. Family support groups provide an avenue for making contact with others in similar situations, who can provide much-needed peer support.

Support Groups

Brain injury *support groups* are a valuable aide to survivors and family caregivers. Support groups are there to assist individuals emotionally and with information until a crisis has passed. They vary from *self-help groups,* where the focus is on personal growth (example: a weight reduction group), to *advocacy groups*, which are community groups that push for social and legislative change (example: MADD – Mothers Against Drunk Drivers). For our purposes here, we will be discussing brain injury support groups.

Many brain injury support groups *do* advocate for the needs of the survivors; for the most part, however, this is a role assumed by provincial/state and national brain injury associations. Support groups are based on the concept that sharing information and personal experiences with others in a similar situation helps individuals cope with a difficult situation. Many communities have separate support groups for survivors and for family members, as their needs differ.

SUPPORT GROUP STRUCTURE

Caregiver support groups generally meet once a month. Some meetings have a guest speaker, or a video providing information on brain injury. This is usually followed by a discussion of the material presented. Some meetings may be more informal and provide a forum for sharing experiences and information. The leadership usually comes from within the group. Health professionals are sometimes called on to create the group and help organize it, but they usually withdraw as leaders after the group is running smoothly. Often professionals are invited to specific meetings and provide related information for group discussion. The group interaction helps relieve family members of their sense of isolation and loneliness.

BENEFITS OF SUPPORT GROUPS

Family support groups can assist family caregivers in at least three ways.

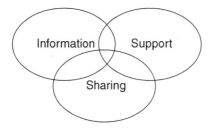

FIGURE 15.1 Components of Support Groups

First, they provide information on the effects of brain injury, on caregiver skills, and on accessing rehabilitation and related community support services. This information may help the family caregiver cope with and adapt to the situation. The family may have received a great deal of information when the survivor was in the acute care hospital and the rehabilitation facility. In fact, sometimes the family receives so much information at this time that it was unable to absorb it all. Now that the survivor is at home, the family may see the need either to acquire additional information, or to review information previously received and determine how it may apply to a particular situation. Table 15.1 lists some topics that may be of interest to a family support group.

Second, support groups provide an opportunity to share experiences, and to learn from others' experiences. This helps reduce feelings of being socially isolated. In our work with families of brain-injured survivors, we found that families living within a relatively small geographic radius often did not know that there were others nearby in the same situation. The demands of caregiving simply did not leave enough time to seek out those others.

The importance of sharing information and experiences was evident in the following example: There was one woman whose husband had suffered a severe brain injury twelve years earlier and another whose husband had suffered a serious injury six months earlier. They did not know each other before they responded to an announcement that a family support group was being formed in their area. The sharing of experiences and emotions, and the support these two women provided each other, helped the younger

TABLE 15.1 Topics for family support groups

Effects of brain injury	Community resources
Management of cognitive	and services
and behavioural problems	Legal issues
Communication: Recognizing	Financial issues
depression/getting help	Recreation and leisure
Impact on the family system	

woman cope with this crisis in her life and demonstrated to the older woman how far she had progressed in her twelve-year journey.

In the process of sharing experiences, established members of the group serve as role models for newer members. The need to learn the caregiver role was expressed this way by a family caregiver in our British Columbia survey: 'I needed help at the time in learning my role as a caregiver and how to accomplish this role. This is also the most common plea I hear from other families and friends of the brain-injured person. "I don't know how to cope with this person – I don't know how to cope."'

A *third* function of family support groups is to offer emotional support during a time of family crisis. Family members can discuss concerns in a safe, accepting, and supportive environment. As one family member stated: 'These meetings provide a place where I am able to unburden myself, learn that I am not alone, and receive support and share experiences.' Emotional support is often needed in dealing with loss and grief.

A brain injury is usually accompanied by many losses, for both the survivor and the family. The survivor may experience loss of memory, physical mobility, and independence, as well as the loss of friends as they drift away after the injury. A family will experience the loss of the son who was; a wife will lose the love of a mate as the husband assumes a more dependent role. Such losses often include threats of additional or future losses; for example, loss of the health of a wage-earning father may lead to loss of income, as well as loss of the father figure in the household. Grief is a response to loss.

There are many theoretical models of grief. Usually these models describe the grief response in terms of stages. The movement between stages does not necessarily follow a particular sequence, and the griever may revisit stages throughout the process. Common to these models are the following stages:

- Shock and disbelief – a sense of numbness, unreality, pain, separation.
- Yearning and protest – feelings of anger.
- Anguish, disorganization, and despair – reality is being recognized; may feel depressed, lonely.
- Reorganization and restitution – gradually grief subsides. Still feel depression but also periods of well-being.

The grieving process requires physical and emotional energy, and usually takes longer than the bereaved anticipates, and much longer than society recognizes. Some people take years to reach the stage of reorganization and restitution, and even then, the pain of the loss may remain for a lifetime. There is no clear end to grief. The bereaved do not forget the past; rather, they gradually learn to live a new life without that which has been lost.

Chronic grief is accumulated or prolonged grief; excessive emotion is demonstrated, and no satisfactory conclusion of the grief is reached. The grieving extends over long periods of time, and new waves of grief are constantly being triggered. The individual with chronic grief has feelings of helplessness, and there is potential for impaired functioning. Chronic grief requires counselling to improve self-confidence and find new direction.

Benefits of Caregiving

Although there are stresses associated with caregiving, there are also rewards. The families of long-term survivors report feelings of happiness when the survivor makes progress. Other positive aspects to caregiving include a sense of fulfilment and an increased appreciation for life in general. The caregiver wife of a brain-injured survivor expressed her feeling this way: 'It's been the greatest challenge of my life and it's taken everything I had to give, but it's worth it. The bond between us is made of steel and will never break. What he has accomplished in his recovery is far more precious to me than the material successes we might have achieved had his injury never occurred.'

Within the group, one will hear family members speak of improvements in the survivor's condition long after the injury occurred. Many caregivers find their greatest reward when their loved one makes progress, no matter how limited. It used to be assumed that all recovery from a brain injury occurred within the first two years of injury, and one may still see this stated in older literature. We now know that *this is simply not true*. Although the primary recovery tends to occur within the first six months after the injury, brain injury survivors continue to make improvements years later. These gains may be limited, but they are victories nonetheless, for both the survivor and the family.

Support groups can be a lifeline to the family caregiver. The caregiver may need to call on friends and relatives to stay with the survivor while attending a group meeting. Most are willing and pleased to assist for a few hours. *Don't be afraid to ask for help!*

Families can inquire about support groups through the nearest Brain Injury Association. See Appendix A for information on these groups.

16. A Second Look

Charles G. Ottewell

This entry to my journal is a follow-up to chapter 3; it was written when I was twenty-seven years old, ten years after my brain injury. I wrote this entry to try and help explain the continuous fight and effort I have and still am battling. I hope this chapter will help whoever reads it to make their transition more understandable as they continue to improve from whatever head injury, brain injury they are recuperating from.

Life is still somewhat of a struggle for me. I still have many of the same *frustrations* which I encountered years ago such as the uncontrolled shakiness in my hands when I get too tired. I'm still walking with a slow gait and a walking-cane, my stamina and physical strength are a lot weaker than normal. My ongoing trouble with not being able to sleep or relax is becoming a more distressful problem for me to try and solve.

I am still *fighting life* everyday, if I may use my old cliché. I'm still trying to understand what has happened to me. Although I have accepted most of my circumstances, I'm still battling with myself. Trying to improve myself so I can leave all my disabilities behind me, which I know *cannot* all be done. But I am learning and teaching

This chapter was previously published in Ottewell, C.G. (1994). 'From the Patient's Point of View.' *Journal of Cognitive Rehabilitation*, 12(3), 8–10. Reprinted with permission.

myself how to cope and to adjust to living with my problems that I encounter day to day.

I'm still only able to mentally and physically take one or two courses a semester at university, which leaves me more than a little discouraged about my progress in working towards a degree in school. I hope to find a career job of some sort for I know I can not change jobs and careers very easily, so it's best I try finding something in a field of work that I like and can handle. After my rugby accident in the spring of 1983, I did not receive any insurance settlements so I am living on a disability pension from the government which pays my rent and not much more. So to save money and pay my enrolment at school is not an easy task, but I do manage somehow.

The obvious and not so obvious stress that I live with day to day: just trying to walk when my left side of my body does not respond to my commands, my hands shaking with ataxia when I get too tired, which makes everyday routines like trying to tie my shoes or pouring a cup of coffee, a demanding task. It is hard for me to accept, when my brain is telling my hands to do something, like to hold a cup still, yet my battle with the ataxia continues on.

Another frustrating reality for me to accept, is that I cannot seem to improve physically. I set up a work-out schedule and exercised actively five days a week for several months, always believing that I could regain some of what I lost in strength and co-ordination, but, with minimal improvements. My walking improved slightly, but there wasn't any other real noticeable improvements. So one of my biggest dreams, just to be able to run a block or even ten feet is as I know for this time of my life unlikely. My brain doesn't seem to allow my body to improve for whatever reason. This is really hard for me to accept and handle, for I've always been an athletic person, and participated in many sports, and I do miss this part of my life. But I know I have to let go of these dreams and try and live as I am now.

One of my major problems early after my accident was to not live in the past. In a sense you have to forget who you once were or what you could do and live and try to be independent and productive as you are now, with whatever disability you have, mine not being able to run or use my hands accurately, mainly my left side of my body does not function accordingly. Now, ten years plus after my accident, I have learned what my brain is capable of and am still trying to re-teach it more.

Your brain can recover some of what you lost prior to your accident, but in my own incident, it has left my left side of my body functioning far from normal, with my leg hyper-extending when I walk, my arm and hand not being very co-ordinated and my left eye weaker, so I have slight double-vision. With lots of work I have been able to re-train my memory and now I can function at quite a high level of intellect.

My level of expectation on myself is so high, I do have a lot of down periods in my life. I feel sorry for myself, my desperation, not doing well enough and wanting to do more, although I think that over time these anxieties have lessened. It is a struggle for me to be completely positive about myself. Always wanting to do more, and manage more, with work and school. I do use up a lot of energy being in these so-called down periods. It does hold me back, but I had and still have to learn how to work through these dark periods of my life. It is still a real struggle for me at times to be positive and feel good and happy about what I have accomplished and what I'm trying to succeed at. I have a tremendous amount of guilt about myself. Not doing as well as other normal peers. With my abilities, I can't keep up to so-called normal people with studying and school and just with everyday activities. It is a big deal to me just to get my left hand to work so it can open the front door. So with my concentration just doing common everyday 'tasks' at times is a major achievement for me.

My Parents

I also have a lot of guilt in how I have affected my family and parents. I'm so sorry for them to have to see me battle with myself and life. One big benefit I had was my parents' support, both my mother and father. I can only try to imagine what their stress has been like since my accident. First, having a healthy seventeen-year-old able-bodied son with future goals ahead of him in his life, then overnight seeing me try and fight to stay alive. From wearing diapers to sitting in a wheelchair. Eventually standing and walking with some difficulty with a cane. They have seen the struggle within myself. Just forcing myself to make the left side of my body function normally, trying to get my left hand to open the door. They get more excited than I do when they see my left arm do a simple routine like carrying a glass of water and not having it spill. They have seen me trip and fall down, but always letting me get up and continue to walk.

Fighting with me to try and keep me active in my studies that last year of school. Having me lash out as I tried to figure out what my capabilities were. Then trying to help me with the confusion I had, to understand my new limitations and my capabilities. Most of my anger and frustrations focused at them, I'm not sure why; and most definitely not warranted. I think I've gone through this period of my recovery for I was and still am trying so hard just to do everyday things. I didn't like myself too much, didn't like having them see me struggle, almost as if I was disappointing to them.

But with my own courage to battle on with life, my parents showed a lot of courage themselves, to let me try, and give me support when I need it. They showed a lot of patience towards me as I tried to continue on with the daily routines of life. They too had to learn with me, just what my capabilities were and could be. They know what my goals are in life, and have seen my failures as well as my successes. In all honesty if my parents hadn't supported me, and showed a great deal of empathy for me, I don't think I would be here today. I'm still entrenched in my daily routines, trying to prove to myself and them that I can contribute and become successful in whatever I decide to do in life.

Life Continues

The first year after my rugby accident I didn't have much of a social life. I only kept a few good friends, who tried to understand my difficult situation. And now being ten years after my accident I have a lot of friends and girlfriends. I had to mature very quickly to understand and try to accept this so-called *new me*. So most of the people I associate with are also more mature and older. I think it is easier meeting people today, for they see me as I am now, walking with a gait and a walking cane, and they didn't know me prior to my accident in 1983. So I don't have to try and be more than what I am doing right now. Just trying to live and being me.

In a lot of ways, I'm also a lot easier to get along with. Understanding my own frustrations that I experience day to day, dealing with my physical disabilities that I encounter with my walking and coordination. I know I'm not the most patient person you've ever met, especially with my own abilities. There is still a lot of uncertainty in my life. Trying to figure out my limitations, and acknowledging my own successes. I feel like I have challenged myself, always trying and wishing I could contribute more. This leaves me more than just a little bit exhausted and worrying about circumstances that I really don't or can't control. Always wanting to do more.

My life is somewhat in limbo right now. I feel thwarted in my attempts in pursuing a job and trying to fulfil my career ambitions. I am extremely frustrated, feeling like I don't have much of a future to look forward to.

I have had limited support from organizations to assist and counsel me towards my long-term goals. The organizations that were, that are supposed to help the brain injured individual at least in my own case, have been of little or no help at all in organizing support for school and/or retraining. I think more funding and proper direction is needed for these groups to become totally useful in the functions in which they were supposed to be intended for. That is, trying to assist the brain injured person with living as independently as possible and succeeding in whatever endeavour they strive for in life. I wish I had had more support, to make my transition in post-secondary education a lot less burdensome, especially financially.

Conclusion

I will admit I'm still somewhat scared every day of my life. Struggling to continue on with life. Being depressed and anxious, waiting for something to happen as I labour with my daily routines. From taking a couple of courses at school to exercising, hoping my strength and walking will improve. I still have many ambitions which I hope to achieve. I feel like I have fought hard to try and minimize a lot of my problems, be it trying to improve my physical abilities or attending college to work towards a degree of some sort. I'm trying not to be so critical of myself and admit my impairments. This has been a very tiring process in my recovery, trying to remain positive, and trying to make a difference in this life. The key words for me are *limitations, acceptance and understanding.* I have become more realistic in what my capabilities are and just what I'm able to do. What I endeavour to do now is work solely with other closed head injury individuals and families and with doctors and therapists and whoever is working with the individual, to help and assist that person succeed and become productive at whatever their goals may be. These goals may be dressing oneself to remembering one's phone number, which as in my own case were tremendous achievements. I know now there is a lot of specific ways to re-train and re-teach a brain-injured person. The process is a lot slower and more patience is needed in order for them to improve and realize what their roles are and how they can become productive in whatever their goals are.

I have worked with a sixteen-year-old boy who is now living with a closed head-injury. My job consisted of helping him with his school work, remembering his home address and phone number and assisting him with daily life skills. I found working with this individual to be very rewarding to see his improvements, but also very frustrating in trying to get more co-operation from the school system and his parents with helping him in his reading and memory troubles. He gained a lot of self-confidence in himself and his abilities. It was also a very positive experience for his self-image and esteem. I felt I made a lot of positive steps forward with this young lad, but he didn't get as much out of it as he could have, for he needed more support. I worked with him just 12 hours per week for 7 months. I know the key to help many brain injured individuals is repetition. I just hope the individual can be counselled to realize just what they are capable of and to try and understand their own circumstances.

Postscript: Charles is now thirty years old, lives independently, and works as a counsellor to persons with closed head injuries.

Appendix A
Resources and Assistance

Brain injury associations are a valuable source of information. Their goal is to improve the quality of life for brain injury survivors and their families. Although the specific objectives of various groups may differ, generally they achieve their goals by providing information about the effects of brain injury and the resources available, as well as advocacy and public and professional education. Information about treatment facilities, rehabilitation, and support groups in your area is available through these associations.

Because the addresses of local associations and support groups change frequently, only the addresses and phone numbers of parent associations are provided. The parent organization will be able to provide you with more detailed information regarding local groups.

CANADA

Canadian Brain Injury Coalition

29 Pearce Avenue
Winnipeg, Manitoba, R2V 2K3
Phone: (204) 334-0471
Fax: (204) 339-1034
Toll free: 1-800-735-CBIC(2242),
e-mail: cbic@pcs.mb.ca

The *Canadian Brain Injury Coalition (CBIC)* facilitates the development of provincial brain injury associations/societies in Canada. The CBIC provides education opportunities regarding brain injury, encourages research, and strives to increase public awareness and understanding about brain injury.

UNITED STATES

The Brain Injury Association, Inc.
(formerly the National Head Injury Foundation, Inc.)

105 North Alfred Street
Alexandria VA 22314
Phone: (703) 236-6000
Fax: (703) 236-6001
Home Page: www.biausa.org
Family Help Line: 1-800-444-6443

The Brain Injury Association (BIA) – originally founded in 1980 as the National Head Injury Foundation is a nonprofit organization encompassing a national network of state associations. The mission of the BIA is to *advocate* for and with people with brain injury, to secure and develop community-based *services* for individuals with brain injury and their families, to support *research* leading to better outcomes that enhance the life of people who sustain a brain injury, and to promote *prevention* of brain injury through public awareness, education, and legislation.

GREAT BRITAIN

Headway National Head Injuries Association

7 King Edward Court
King Edward Street
Nottingham, England NG1 1EW
Phone: (0115) 912 1000
Fax: (0115) 912 1011

Headway originated in 1979 in response to the growing number of people surviving severe head injuries. Presently affiliated are 110 locally organized self-help groups. These groups exist throughout the United Kingdom, with five groups in Ireland.

Headway's work involves:

1. Giving support to the head-injured person and to relatives, carers, and friends.
2. Helping in the rehabilitation of the head-injured person at home.
3. Providing and encouraging social, leisure, and other activities.
4. Arranging opportunities for those involved to meet and share their experiences and concerns.
5. Pressing for improvement in national and local services for the head injured.

NEW ZEALAND

Head Injury Society of New Zealand

Office address:
Head Injury Society of New Zealand Inc.
5th Floor, Rossmore House
123 Molesworth St.
Wellington, New Zealand
Phone: (04) 472-2977
Fax: (04) 499-8854
Home Page: http://www.head~injury.org.nz/
Postal address:
PO Box 12–245
Wellington, New Zealand

The mission of the society is to strive for a quality of life that maximizes potential, choice, and independence for people with head injury, their families, and caregivers.

AUSTRALIA

The Head Injury Council of Australia (HICOA)

There are seven affiliate bodies: Queensland, New South Wales, Victoria, Northern Territory, Tasmania, South Australia, and Western Australia.

Contact:
Head Injury Society of Western Australia Inc.
645 Canning Highway
Alfred Cove, WA 6154
PO Box 298, Applecross, WA 6154
Phone: (09) 330-6370
Fax: (09) 317-2264

INTERNET

Website addresses are changing almost daily. We are listing a few
that are current at the time of publication:

http://www.neuroskills.com/~cns/tbi/injury.html
Home page of the Centre for Neuro Skills, Bakerfield, CA, and Irv-
ing, Texas

http://www.sasquatch.com/tbi/
The home page of the Perspective Network ABI/TBI Information
Project.

http://mars.ark.com/~headstrt/
One of the selections listed (tbikids.htm) provides a chatline for
teens and kids.

Listserv

Listservs are formed to provide a means of discussion on a particular
topic. *Tbi-sprt* was created for the exchange of information by survivors, supporters, and professionals concerned with traumatic brain
injury and other neurological impairments. To subscribe, send an
e-mail message to:

listserv@sjuvm.stjohns.edu

with this message:

Subscribe TBI-SPRT (your name)

Appendix B
Glossary

Abstract: Refers to concepts that may be difficult to understand; concepts that are theoretical or detached, dealing with things that cannot actually be seen. Some patients with cognitive deficits can only understand concepts that are 'concrete,' or related to something tangible in the environment.

Amnesia: Loss of memory, either partial or total; functional inability to recall the personal past.

Anticonvulsants: Medications that prevent or relieve epileptic seizures. A person may be placed on such medications as a precaution against seizures, or the medication may be administered to halt a lengthy seizure.

Apathy: A lack of interest or concern.

Aphasia: Loss of the ability to express oneself and/or to understand language. Aphasia may be either sensory or receptive (in which language is not understood), or expressive, or motor (in which words cannot be formed or expressed). Sensory aphasia affects specific language functions, as in DYSLEXIA or ALEXIA. Expressive aphasia may be complete, as in DYSPHASIA (in which speech is impaired), or as in AGRAPHIA (in which writing is affected). Often the condition is a mixture of both expressive and receptive aphasia.

Receptive aphasia: Refers to an inability to understand what someone else is saying. This is often associated with damage to the left temporal area of the brain.

Expressive aphasia: Refers to an inability to express oneself. Some patients may know what they want to say but may not be able to form the words. Other patients may be able to form the words but many of the words they say may not 'make sense.' Expressive aphasia is often associated with the left frontal area of the brain.

Ataxia: Inability to co-ordinate muscle movements, or having irregular muscle movements. This can interfere with the person's ability to walk, talk, eat, perform self-care tasks, and work.

Brain injury: Injury to the brain tissue (inside the skull), resulting in damage or the brain's inability to function properly.

Traumatic brain injury: Injury to the brain caused by a trauma, such as a car accident, fall, or sporting injury.

Acquired brain injury: The name given to both traumatic brain injuries and those caused by stroke or by a broken blood vessel that causes bleeding into the brain tissue.

Brain stem: The lower portion of the brain, which connects the brain to the spinal column. The brain stem co-ordinates the body's vital functions (breathing, blood pressure, and pulse). It also houses the reticular formation, which controls consciousness, drowsiness, and attention.

Cerebellum: The portion of the brain located below the cortex. The cerebellum is concerned with co-ordinating movements.

Cognition: Embracing all forms of knowing, including perceiving, imagining, reasoning, and judging.

Coma: Unconsciousness lasting for more than a brief period of time. A state of unconsciousness where the person cannot be aroused and/or does not respond.

Disorientation: Not knowing where you are, who you are, or the time. Often professionals use the term 'oriented in all three spheres,' or, 'oriented times three,' which refers to person, place, and time.

Edema: Collection of fluid causing swelling; this can happen in the brain.

Frontal lobe: The area of the brain located at the front of the brain on the left and right sides. This area plays a role in controlling emotions, motivation, social skills, and speech, and in inhibiting impulses. The 'executive functions' are also located here; these include the ability to plan and to carry out activities.

Frustration tolerance: The ability to deal with frustrating events in daily life; there will be a point at which the person can no longer control his or her anger in a situation. (May respond by yelling, throwing things, or becoming aggressive).

Hemorrhage: Bleeding that may occur following trauma. Bleeding may occur within the brain when blood vessels in the skull or the brain are damaged.

Incontinence: Inability to control bowel and/or bladder functions.

Memory: The process of perceiving information, organizing and storing it, and retrieving it at a later time as needed. Memory is a complex function that involves many parts of the brain working together. There are different 'types' of memory, including immediate (repeating a phone number), recent (recalling what occurred the previous day), and remote (recalling the name of a childhood friend).

Motor control: Regulation of the timing and amount of contraction of muscles of the body to produce smooth, co-ordinated movement. The regulation is carried out by operation of the nervous system.

Fine motor control: Delicate movements as in writing or playing the piano.

Gross motor control: Large, strong movements as in chopping wood or walking.

Labile or **Lability**: Unpredictable mood swings from tears to laughter; these are uncontrollable and may not reflect the underlying feeling.

Occipital lobe: The posterior (back) part of each side of the brain, involved in perceiving and understanding visual information.

Parietal lobe: The upper and middle lobes of each side of the brain, involved in perceiving and understanding sensations (e.g., touch, heat, cold). The right side is also responsible for perception functions (e.g., the ability of the brain to interpret information received through the senses); the left side has important language functions.

Post-trauma amnesia (PTA): The time between injury and recovery of full memory for day-to-day events. The length of PTA is regarded as an indicator of eventual recovery.

Temporal lobe: The lower middle part of each side of the brain, concerned with sound interpretation and perception, and important for hearing as well as the control of behaviour.

Tracheostomy: A surgical opening at the front of the throat providing access to the trachea (windpipe) to allow breathing.

Appendix C
Suggestions for Further Reading

There are many books and articles about brain injury and about caregiving. You may find useful information in the caregiving literature, even if the book or article is directed toward a chronic condition other than brain injury. Some books and articles may be found in your local public library or local bookstore. Search the following subjects: caregiving, brain injury, head injury. Additional books and articles of a more academic nature may be found at your local university library (sample journal articles listed below). The list provided here is only a sample of the reading material available; additional information is becoming available daily. Many local brain injury associations (see Appendix A for a listing) provide a library on the effects of brain injury. Many of these associations also publish their own newsletters and other materials.

Lay Caregiving/Personal Story Books:

Carter, R., & Golant, S.K. (1994). *Helping Yourself Help Others: A book for Caregivers.* New York: Times Books.

Gronwell, D., Wrighton, P., & Waddell, P. (1990). *Head injury: The Facts – A Guide for Families and Care-givers.* Oxford: Oxford University Press.

Hughes, B.K. (1990). *Parenting a Child with Traumatic Brain Injury.* Springfield, Ill.: Charles C. Thomas Publishers.

Krieg, M. (1995). *Awake Again.* Santa Cruz, Calif.: KM Publishing.

Locke, S.A. (1994). *Coping with Loss: A Guide for Caregivers.* Springfield, Ill.: C.C. Thomas.

Mace, N.L., & Rabins, P.V. (1991). *The 36-hour Day*. Baltimore, MD: The Johns Hopkins University Press.

Maxwell, M.C. (1988). *Missing Pieces: Mending the Head Injury Family*. Fort Colins, Co.: Brain Technologies Corp.

Singer, George H.S., Glang, A., & Williams, J.M. (1996). *Children with Acquired Brain Injury: Educating and Supporting Families*. Baltimore, Md.: Paul H. Brookes.

Slater, B. (1984). *Stranger in My Bed*. New York: Arbor House.

Williams, J.M., & Kay, T. (eds.) (1991). *Head Injury: A Family Matter*. Baltimore, Md.: Paul H. Brookes.

Professional Journal Articles and Books:

Acorn, S. (1993). 'Head Injured Survivors: Caregivers and Support Groups.' *Journal of Advanced Nursing, 18*, 39–45.

Anthony, P., & McGill, J. (eds.). (1994). (Special issue devoted to persons with brain injury and leisure implications.) *Journal of Leisurability, 21*(2).

Barga, N.K., (1996). 'Students with Learning Disabilities in Education: Managing a Disability. *Journal of Learning Disabilities 29*, (4) 413–21.

Batshaw, M.L., & Perret, Y.M. (1992). (eds). *Children with Disabilities: A Medical Primer* (3rd). Baltimore, Md.: Paul H. Brookes.

Broman, S.H., & Michel, M.E. (eds) (1995). *Traumatic Head Injury in Children*. New York: Oxford University Press.

Brooks, D.N. (1991). 'The Head Injured Family.' *Journal of Clinical and Experimental Neuropsychology, 13* (1), 155–88.

Chwalisz, K. (1992). 'Perceived Stress and Caregiver Burden After Brain Injury: A Theoretical Integration.' *Rehabilitation Psychology, 37* (3), 189–203.

Clements, C.B. (1994). *The Arts/fitness Quality of Life Activities Program: Creative Ideas for Working with Older Adults in Group Settings*. Baltimore, Md.: Health Professions Press.

Florian, V., Katz, S., & Lahav, V. (1989). 'Impact of Traumatic Brain Damage on Family Dynamics and Functioning: A Review.' *Brain Injury, 3* (3), 219–33.

Hutchison, P., & McGill, J. (1992). *Leisure, Integration and Community*. Concord, Ont.: Leisurability Publications.

Kraus, J.F., Rock, A., & Hemyari, P. (1990). 'Brain Injuries Among Infants, Children, Adolescents and Young Adults.' *American Journal of Diseases of Children, 144*, 684–91.

Lezak, M. (1988). 'Brain Damage Is a Family Affair.' *Journal of Clinical and Experimental Neuropsychology, 10* (1), 111–23.

Livingston, M.G., & Brooks, D.N. (1988). 'The Burden on Families of the Brain Injured: A Review.' *Journal of Head Trauma Rehabilitation, 3* (4), 6–15.

Novack, T.A., Bergquist, T.F., Bennett, G., & Gouvier, W.D. (1991). 'Primary Caregiver Distress Following Severe Head Injury.' *Journal of Head Trauma Rehabilitation, 6* (4), 69–77.

Rosenthal, M., Griffith, M.R., Bond, M.R., & Miller, J.D. (eds). (1990). *Rehabilitation of the Adult and Child with Traumatic Brain Injury.* Philadelphia: F.A. Davis.

Schulz, R., Visintainer, P., & Williamson, G.M. (1990). 'Psychiatric and Physical Morbidity Effects of Caregiving.' *Journal of Gerontology: Psychological Studies, 45*, 181–91.

Wexler, D. (1991). *The Adolescent Self: Strategies for Self-management, Self-soothing, and Self-esteem in Adolescents.* New York: W.W. Norton.

Whitehouse, A.M., & Carey, J.L. (1991). 'Composition and Concerns of a Support Group for Families of Individuals with Brain Injury. *Journal of Cognitive Rehabilitation*, 26–9.

Zeigler, E.A. (1987). 'Spouses of Persons Who Are Brain Injured: Overlooked Victims.' *Journal of Rehabilitation, 53* (1), 50–3.

Contributors

Sonia Acorn, RN, PhD
Associate Professor
School of Nursing
The University of British Columbia
T 301 – 2211 Wesbrook Mall
Vancouver, British Columbia
V6T 2B5

David Blanche, BRe
Counsellor/Therapist
931 – 6th St.
New Westminster
Vancouver, British Columbia
V3L 3C8

Carroll O. David, MSSW
Director of Family Services
Tangram Rehabilitation Network
220 West Hutchison St.
San Marcos, Texas
73666

Claudia Berwald, MSW, RSW
Professional Services Social
Work/Adult Brain Injury Program
Glenrose Rehabilitation Hospital
10230 – 111 Ave.
Edmonton, Alberta
T5G 0B7

Rick Brown, MSW, RSW
Professional Services Social
Work/Adult Brain Injury Program
Glenrose Rehabilitation Hospital
10230 – 111 Ave.
Edmonton, Alberta
T5G 0B7

John Higenbottam, PhD, CHE
Vice President
Clinical Services
Continuing Care, Psychiatry,
Rehabilitation CPUs
Vancouver Hospital & Health
Sciences Centre
Vancouver, British Columbia
V5Z 2G1

Patrick Hirschi, MSW, RSW
Professional Services Social
Work/Adult Brain Injury
Program
Glenrose Rehabilitation Hospital
10230 – 111 Ave.
Edmonton, Alberta
T5G 0B7

Charles Killingsworth, PhD, CTRS
Professor, Department of Health,
Phy. Ed. & Recreation
School of Education
Pittsburg State University
1701 S. Broadway, Pittsburg
Kansas 66762–7557

Penny Offer, MSW, MPA
Program Director
Adolescent/Young Adult
G.F. Strong Rehabilitation Centre
4255 Laurel St.
Vancouver, British Columbia
V5Z 2G9

Charles G. Ottewell
Rehabilitation Therapy
Consultant for the Traumatically
Brain Injured
218 – 3896 Laurel St.
Burnaby, British Columbia
V5G 4C7

Mary Pepping, PhD
Clinical Psychology and
Neuropsychology
413 Thirty-First Ave.
Seattle, WA
98122– 6319

J. David Seaton
Executive Director
Tangram Rehabilitation Network
220 West Hutchison St.
San Marcos, Texas
78666

John Simpson
Simpson Rehab Management
99 – 46511 Chilliwack Lake Road
Sardis, British Columbia
V2R 3S4

Anne Sulzberger, Dip RT
Deep Cove Recreation Therapy
Services
4352 Strathcona Rd.
North Vancouver, British Columbia
V7G 1G3

Marilyn Unger, PhD
Adolescent/Young Adult Program
G.F. Strong Rehabilitation Centre
4255 Laurel St.
Vancouver, British Columbia
V5Z 2G9

R. Brian Webster, BA, LLB
R.B. Webster & Associates
Barristers & Solicitors
#600 North Tower
5811 Cooney Rd.
Richmond, British Columbia
V6X 3M1